Reproductive Ethics

ISSUES

Volume 178

Series Editor

Lisa Firth

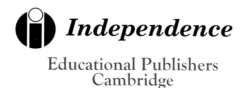

Independence

Educational Publishers
Cambridge

First published by Independence
The Studio, High Green
Great Shelford
Cambridge CB22 5EG
England

© Independence 2009

British Library Cataloguing in Publication Data
Reproductive Ethics — (Issues; v. 178)
1. Human reproductive technology — moral and ethical aspects
I. Series II. Firth, Lisa
176-dc22

ISBN-13: 978 1 86168 502 5 ⊙

Printed in Great Britain
MWL Print Group Ltd

Cover
The illustration on the front cover is by
Angelo Madrid.

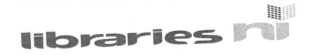

CONTENTS

Chapter One: Making Babies

Chapter Two: Ethical Dilemmas

Useful information for readers

Dear Reader,

Issues: Reproductive Ethics

Since the birth of the first 'test-tube baby' over 30 years ago, society has witnessed a revolution in the area of artificial reproduction. However, many of the options open to infertile people also have ethical implications. This title examines the issues surrounding IVF, egg and embryo freezing, donor insemination and surrogacy, as well as the creation of so-called 'saviour siblings' and 'designer babies' and the use of embryos in research.

The purpose of *Issues*

Reproductive Ethics is the one hundred and seventy-eighth volume in the **Issues** series. The aim of this series is to offer up-to-date information about important issues in our world. Whether you are a regular reader or new to the series, we do hope you find this book a useful overview of the many and complex issues involved in the topic.

Titles in the **Issues** series are resource books designed to be of especial use to those undertaking project work or requiring an overview of facts, opinions and information on a particular subject, particularly as a prelude to undertaking their own research.

The information in this book is not from a single author, publication or organisation; the value of this unique series lies in the fact that it presents information from a wide variety of sources, including:

⇨ Government reports and statistics
⇨ Newspaper articles and features
⇨ Information from think-tanks and policy institutes
⇨ Magazine features and surveys
⇨ Website material
⇨ Literature from lobby groups and charitable organisations.*

Critical evaluation

Because the information reprinted here is from a number of different sources, readers should bear in mind the origin of the text and whether the source is likely to have a particular bias or agenda when presenting information (just as they would if undertaking their own research). It is hoped that, as you read about the many aspects of the issues explored in this book, you will critically evaluate the information presented. It is important that you decide whether you are being presented with facts or opinions. Does the writer give a biased or an unbiased report? If an opinion is being expressed, do you agree with the writer?

Reproductive Ethics offers a useful starting point for those who need convenient access to information about the many issues involved. However, it is only a starting point. Following each article is a URL to the relevant organisation's website, which you may wish to visit for further information.

Kind regards,

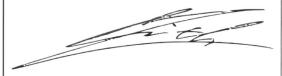

Lisa Firth
Editor, **Issues** series

** Please note that Independence Publishers has no political affiliations or opinions on the topics covered in the **Issues** series, and any views quoted in this book are not necessarily those of the publisher or its staff.*

ISSUES TODAY
A RESOURCE FOR KEY STAGE 3

Younger readers can also benefit from the thorough editorial process which characterises the **Issues** series with our resource books for 11- to 14-year-old students, **Issues Today**. In addition to containing information from a wide range of sources, rewritten with this age group in mind, **Issues Today** titles also feature comprehensive glossaries, an accessible and attractive layout and handy tasks and assignments which can be used in class, for homework or as a revision aid. In addition, these titles are fully photocopiable. For more information, please visit our website (www.independence.co.uk).

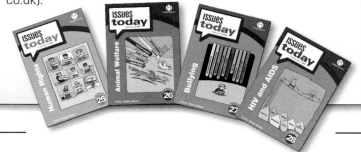

Doing without sex

Will there come a day when reproduction is entirely separated from the human body?

Pregnancy and childbirth are major challenges to the female body. An expectant mother has to provide nutrition and a safe environment for her growing baby, and childbirth thrusts a vulnerable baby into a harsh outside world. Until recently, death of mother or infant during or immediately after birth was common in the West (and remains so in many parts of the developing world).

Much science fiction includes visions of pregnancy outside the human body

Small wonder, then, that much science fiction includes visions of pregnancy outside the human body. In Aldous Huxley's *Brave New World*, for example, babies are grown in special incubators and reproduction is entirely divorced from sex. This has the advantage that the authorities can control what type of child is

wellcometrust

produced, from the 'alpha' elite to the 'deltas' and 'epsilons' who do manual work.

In vitro fertilisation

The first step in producing a new individual, fertilisation, can take place outside the body. In 1978, Louise Brown became the world's first 'test-tube baby'. Sperm and egg are fused in culture; the embryo develops a short while and is then implanted into the mother's womb.

This procedure, in vitro fertilisation (IVF), has become routine, and around two million children have been born by IVF.

It is used when would-be parents have difficulty conceiving a child. For example, an egg may not travel

through a woman's reproductive system properly or a man may have a low sperm count. If a man has immotile sperm, which cannot swim to an egg, a sperm nucleus can be directly injected into the egg (a procedure known as intracytoplasmic sperm injection, ICSI).

Although common, in vitro fertilisation still has a relatively low success rate (typically about 20 per cent) and is not a pleasant experience. It is far from a 'lifestyle' option but a last chance for couples having difficulties conceiving.

The artificial womb

Creating an embryo may be relatively easy but nurturing it to the point of independent existence certainly is not. The arrival of artificial wombs has made headlines periodically over the past decade, but they remain science fiction at the moment.

The medical need arises from the desire to save developing fetuses that might otherwise die – for example, if an expectant mother's womb is damaged in a road traffic accident. A second important area is the survival of premature babies. Great strides have been made in this area, and infants born so prematurely that they would have died in previous eras can often be saved. But there is a limit and even those that do survive often suffer brain damage or other harm.

The growth of a new baby in the womb is highly complex, and the placenta plays a key role in providing the right nutrients, protecting the fetus from harmful substances and removing waste products. Recreating these functions artificially is a huge challenge.

One approach is to try to grow womb-like structures in culture. A group at Cornell University in the

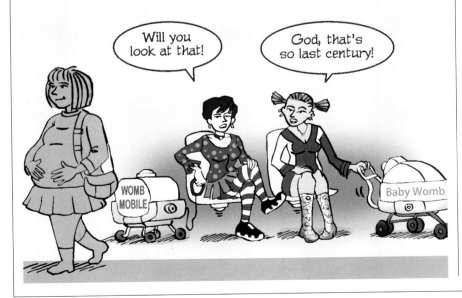

USA has had some success in growing cells from the lining of a human uterus and is using tissue engineering to mould them into a womb shape. They have also grown mouse embryos nearly to term in an artificial womb (though the newborn mice did not survive).

In separate experiments, a Japanese team has used 'uterine tanks' to support the development of goat fetuses. They took early stage embryos from pregnant goats and brought them to full term (though again the newborn animals did not survive).

Medical need and social application

This kind of work inevitably seems to lead people to imagine 'baby factories' growing new infants to order. In *Brave New World*, the State was the bad guy, seeking central control, but now the fears are more about individuals creating 'super-babies' or babies becoming commodities chosen to order like a new car.

But it is worth remembering that the primary purpose of this research is to save babies' lives or to help the infertile. There may one day be a possibility for wider application of these technologies, but for the foreseeable future these are likely to be difficult procedures to carry out and used only when absolutely necessary.

Take preimplantation genetic diagnosis (PGD). This involves taking a cell from an early human embryo during IVF and carrying out genetic tests on it. Through this technique, parents at risk of having a boy with an X-linked genetic disease can have a female embryo implanted. Or in families with inherited disorders, an embryo without a disease gene can be implanted.

There are fears that this could be used to create 'designer babies', where parents select embryos with particular features. In reality, the links between genes and particular features (intelligence, say) are so complicated that this is unlikely to be a realistic scenario. Then the procedures themselves are difficult and not undertaken lightly. Finally, in the UK at least, reproductive technologies are highly regulated (by the Human Fertilisation and Embryology Authority), so socially undesirable applications would face many hurdles.

⇨ The above information is reprinted with kind permission from the Wellcome Trust. Visit www.wellcome.ac.uk for more information on this and other related topics.

© Big Picture Publications

Fertility problems

What are they?

If you and your partner have been diagnosed as having fertility problems, it means you've been trying for a baby for at least a year without success. It doesn't mean you'll never be able to have a baby. There are no guarantees, but there are treatments that can help.

In the UK, about one in seven couples seek medical help to have a baby

If you've been trying for a baby for at least a year, your doctor may suggest some tests to find out what the problem is. You can get help whether or not you've had a child before.[1]

Being unable to have a baby is hard to cope with. Tests and treatments for infertility can be a strain, both physically and emotionally. It may help you and your partner to talk to a special counsellor.

Key points about infertility
⇨ Infertility is very common. In the UK, about one in seven couples seek medical help to have a baby.[2]
⇨ The most common causes in women are ovulation problems and damaged or blocked tubes.
⇨ The most common causes in men are a low sperm count and poor-quality sperm.
⇨ In up to one-third of infertile couples, doctors can't find a reason for the infertility.
⇨ To improve your chances of getting pregnant, you should have sex every two or three days.[1]
⇨ If you're a woman aged 35 or older and you're having problems getting pregnant, don't wait more than a year before you go for help. Many treatments don't work so well when a woman is older.

How you get pregnant
It's useful to know a little about how a pregnancy normally begins. This can help you understand what can go wrong.

To get pregnant:

⇨ The woman has to produce an egg;
⇨ The man has to produce healthy sperm;
⇨ The egg has to travel from the woman's ovary into her fallopian tube;
⇨ The sperm have to swim up through the vagina and womb, into the fallopian tube to meet the egg;
⇨ The egg has to be fertilised by the man's sperm;
⇨ The fertilised egg has to travel down the fallopian tube and embed (plant itself) in the woman's womb.

More than eight in ten couples trying to get pregnant are successful within one year. And more than nine in ten couples get pregnant within two years.[1]

How egg and sperm join together
When a man ejaculates inside a woman, one of his sperm may fertilise the egg. Here is what happens:[3]
⇨ The man's semen (containing sperm) gets pushed up into the vagina;
⇨ About one per cent of sperm (that's about 400,000) swim up to the

cervix, the neck of the womb. The rest die or fall out f the vagina;

⇨ If a woman is in her fertile period, the mucus is thin and watery, helping the sperm swim up to the fallopian tubes;

⇨ If there is an egg inside one of the tubes, the sperm try to push through the egg wall;

⇨ The first one through will fertilise the egg;

⇨ The genes from the egg and sperm combine inside a single cell.

After fertilisation

⇨ The fertilised egg moves down the fallopian tube to the womb. This takes several days.

⇨ It starts growing and embeds in the lining of the womb, called the endometrium.

⇨ Now it's called an embryo. It forms the placenta to get food from its mother. It's only at this stage that pregnancy has started.

⇨ The placenta makes a special hormone to make the lining of the womb thicken. The hormone also prevents the woman having her period.

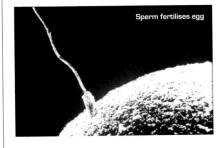
Sperm fertilises egg

When to have sex

A woman is most likely to get pregnant (most fertile) from four or five days before she ovulates until up to a few hours afterwards. This is the likeliest time that the sperm will fertilise an egg.

Many couples who are trying for a baby concentrate on having sex around this time. There are various ways you can work this out. Some women use special hormone kits from a pharmacy. Other women take their temperature or check the fluid in their vagina. This fluid tends to be thin and stretchy when she is fertile.

Still, it's easy to miss the most fertile time of the month. The length of a woman's menstrual cycle can vary and some women ovulate earlier in their cycle than others. So it's very

difficult to be precise, even if you are using hormone kits. Having sex by the calendar can also be stressful and disappointing.

For these reasons, doctors usually advise couples not to try to have sex at certain times of the month, but instead to have sex every two to three days.[1] That way, you're less likely to miss the time that you are ovulating.

What can go wrong

There are many reasons why a couple may find it hard to get pregnant. Either or both partners may have a problem that doctors can identify with tests.

⇨ In two in ten infertile couples, the man has a problem.

⇨ In about four in ten, the woman does.

⇨ In a further three in ten or four in ten, both partners have a problem.

Sometimes, doctors can't work out why you're finding it hard to get pregnant. This is called unexplained infertility.

Problems getting pregnant: the woman

Here are the most common problems that stop a woman getting pregnant:[4]

⇨ Problems ovulating;

⇨ Early menopause;

⇨ Low hormone levels;

⇨ Damaged or blocked tubes;

⇨ Endometriosis;

⇨ Fibroids.

Problems getting pregnant: the man

Here are the most common reasons why men have fertility problems:[4,5]

⇨ Problems with sperm;

⇨ Problems getting sperm to the right place;

⇨ Sperm antibodies.

Why us?

Things that lower your chances of getting pregnant are called risk factors. Here are the main risk factors for infertility:

⇨ Getting older;

⇨ Smoking, alcohol and drugs;

⇨ Being overweight or underweight;

⇨ Testicles are too warm;

⇨ Illness;

Glossary

Ejaculation
When a man ejaculates, his penis suddenly releases semen, the white or transparent fluid that carries sperm.

Genes
Your genes are the parts of your cells that contain instructions for how your body works. Genes are found on chromosomes, structures that sit in the nucleus at the middle of each of your cells. You have 23 pairs of chromosomes in your normal cells, each of which has thousands of genes. You get one set of chromosomes, and all of the genes that are on them, from each of your parents.

⇨ Radiation or dangerous chemicals.

References

1 National Institute for Clinical Excellence. *Fertility: Assessment and treatment for people with fertility problems.* August 2003. Available at http://www.nice.org.uk/pdf/CG011niceguideline.pdf (accessed on 13 June 2008).

2 Cahill DJ, Wardle PG. Management of infertility. *BMJ.* 2002; 325: 28-32.

3 Meniru GI. Fertilization, implantation and early development. In: *Cambridge guide to infertility management and assisted reproduction.* Cambridge University Press, Cambridge, UK; 2001.

4 Meniru GI. Evaluation of the infertile couple. In: *Cambridge guide to infertility management and assisted reproduction.* Cambridge University Press, Cambridge, UK; 2001.

5 Wong WY, Thomas CM, Merkus JM, et al. Male factor subfertility: possible causes and the impact of nutritional factors. *Fertility and Sterility.* 2000; 73: 435-442.

⇨ The above information is reprinted with kind permission from the BMJ Publishing Group. Visit www.bmj.com for more information.

Causes of infertility

Infertility can be caused by many different factors and, in 30% of couples, a cause cannot be identified

Infertility in women

Ovulation disorders

Infertility is most commonly caused by problems with ovulation (the monthly release of an egg). Some of these problems stop women releasing eggs at all, and some cause an egg to be released during some cycles, but not others. Ovulation problems can occur as a result of a number of conditions that are outlined below.

⇨ Premature ovarian failure – when your ovaries stop working before the age of 40.

⇨ Polycystic ovary syndrome (PCOS) – a condition which makes it more difficult for the ovaries to produce an egg.

Women in their early twenties are about twice as fertile as women in their late thirties

---

⇨ Thyroid problems – both an overactive and an underactive thyroid can prevent ovulation.

⇨ Chronic conditions – if you have a debilitating condition, such as cancer or AIDS, it can prevent your ovaries from releasing eggs.

Womb and fallopian tubes

The fallopian tubes transport an egg from the ovary to the womb, where the fertilised egg will grow. If the womb or fallopian tubes become damaged or stop working, then it may be very difficult to conceive naturally. This can occur following a number of procedures or conditions, as outlined below:

⇨ Pelvic surgery – this can sometimes cause damage and scarring to the fallopian tubes.

⇨ Cervical surgery – this can sometimes cause scarring, or shorten the cervix (neck of the womb).

⇨ Submucosal fibroids – are benign (non-cancerous) tumours that develop in the muscle underneath the inner lining of the womb, and may prevent implantation.

⇨ Endometriosis – this is a condition where cells, normally found in the womb lining, start growing on other organs. This can cause adhesions in the pelvis and limit the movement of the fimbria (tiny fronds at the end of the fallopian tubes) which direct the egg into the tube.

⇨ Previous sterilisation – some women choose to be sterilised if they do not wish to have any more children. Sterilisation involves blocking the fallopian tubes to make it impossible for an egg to travel to the womb. This process is rarely reversible. If you do have a sterilisation reversed, it will not necessarily mean that you will become fertile again.

Medicines and drugs

The side effects of some types of medication and drugs can affect your fertility. These medicines are outlined below.

⇨ Non-steroidal anti-inflammatory drugs (NSAIDs) – long-term use or a high dosage of NSAIDs like ibuprofen or aspirin can make it more difficult to conceive.

⇨ Chemotherapy – the medicines used with chemotherapy can sometimes cause ovarian failure, which means your ovaries will no longer be able to function properly. Ovarian failure can be permanent.

⇨ Illegal drugs – drugs such as marijuana and cocaine can seriously affect your fertility, making it more difficult to ovulate. They may also adversely affect the functioning of your fallopian tubes.

Age

Infertility in women is also linked to age. Women in their early twenties are about twice as fertile as women in their late thirties. The biggest decrease in fertility begins during the mid thirties.

Infertility in men

Semen

The most common cause of male infertility is abnormal semen (the fluid ejaculated during sex that contains sperm). Abnormal semen accounts for 75% of male infertility

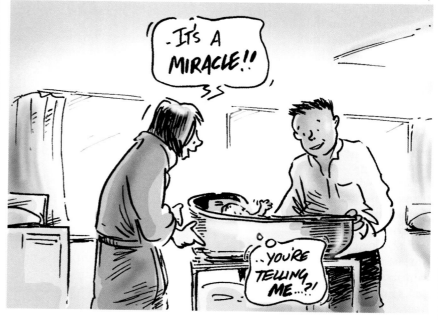

cases, and the cause of abnormal semen is often unknown. Semen can be abnormal for a number of reasons which are outlined below:

- ⇨ Decreased number of sperm – you may have a very low sperm count, or have no sperm at all.
- ⇨ Decreased sperm mobility – if you have decreased sperm mobility, it will be harder for your sperm to swim to the egg.
- ⇨ Abnormal sperm – sometimes sperm can be an abnormal shape, making it harder for them to move and fertilise an egg.

Many cases of abnormal semen are unexplained, but there are several factors which can affect semen and sperm.

Testicles

The testicles are responsible for producing and storing sperm. If they are damaged, it can seriously affect the quality of your semen. This may occur if you have:

- ⇨ an infection of your testicles;
- ⇨ testicular cancer; or,
- ⇨ have undergone testicular surgery.

Ejaculation disorders

Some men have a condition which makes it difficult for them to ejaculate. For example, retrograde ejaculation, causes you to ejaculate semen into your bladder. The ejaculatory ducts can also sometimes become blocked, or obstructed, and this too can make it difficult to ejaculate normally.

Medicines and drugs

- ⇨ Sulfasalazine – this is an anti-inflammatory medicine used to treat conditions such as Crohn's disease (inflammation of the intestine) and rheumatoid arthritis (painful swelling of the joints). This medicine can decrease your number of sperm. However, its effects are only temporary, and your sperm count should return to normal when you stop taking it.
- ⇨ Anabolic steroids – these steroids are often used illegally to build muscles and improve athletic performance. Long-term use, or abuse, of anabolic steroids can reduce your sperm count and sperm mobility.
- ⇨ Chemotherapy – the medicines used with chemotherapy can sometimes severely reduce the production of sperm.

Factors that affect both men and women

There are a number of factors that can affect fertility in both men and women. These include:

- ⇨ Weight – being overweight, or obese, reduces both male and female fertility. In women, it can affect ovulation. Being underweight can also impact on fertility, particularly for women, who will not ovulate if they are severely underweight.
- ⇨ Sexually transmitted infections (STIs) – there are several STIs which can cause infertility. The most common is chlamydia, which can damage the fallopian tubes in women and cause swelling and tenderness of the scrotum (pouch of skin containing the testes) in men.
- ⇨ Smoking – not only does smoking affect your general and long-term health, it can also affect fertility.
- ⇨ Occupational and environmental factors – exposure to certain pesticides, metals and solvents can affect fertility in both men and women.
- ⇨ Stress – if either you or your partner are stressed, it may affect your relationship. Stress can reduce libido (sexual desire), therefore reducing the frequency of sexual intercourse. Severe stress may also affect female ovulation and can limit sperm production.

⇨ The above information is reprinted with kind permission from NHS Choices. Visit www.nhs.uk for more information.

IVF: the birth that started a revolution

As the world's first test-tube baby reaches 30, Judith Woods investigates how family life has been changed by science

By Judith Woods

Thirty years ago this week Louise Brown, the first test-tube baby, was born, and the world of fertility changed forever. Her mother, Lesley, 33, had blocked fallopian tubes, so Patrick Steptoe and Robert Edwards took an egg from one of her ovaries, under anaesthetic, and fertilised it with sperm from her husband, John, in a laboratory, before placing it in her uterus. Nine months later, on 25 July 1978, Louise was delivered by Caesarean section at Oldham and District General Hospital.

Since that day, a series of in-vitro fertilisation (IVF) breakthroughs has enabled tens of thousands of British couples to have the children they longed for. Other leaps have included treatments for male infertility, the use of donor eggs, surrogates and the genetic screening of embryos. In Britain alone, 111,633 children have been born through fertility treatment; worldwide, the figure is estimated to be 3.5 million. The latest figures from the Human Fertilisation and Embryology Authority (HFEA), the regulatory body set up in 1991, show that 32,626 couples in Britain had IVF in 2005, leading to a total – including twins and triplets – of

11,262 children. About 25 per cent of IVF treatments are funded by the NHS; the rest are paid for privately, costing up to £8,000 a cycle.

But while IVF has answered the prayers of many couples, it is not a cure-all. The average success rate nationally for women under 35 is 29.6 per cent, while those aged between 40-42 have just a ten per cent chance of conceiving using their own eggs. (There are exceptions: at the Assisted Reproduction and Gynaecology Centre in London, for example, the take-home baby rate is 59.9 per cent for women under 35.)

And fertility treatments are also transforming the British family, raising ethical questions about concepts such as 'saviour siblings', babies genetically matched and created to provide tissue – often umbilical cord stem cells – to treat disease in an older child. Similarly, treatment for post-menopausal women, same-sex couples and the spectres of sex selection for social reasons (illegal in the UK) and 'designer babies', where embryos are chosen or discarded for reasons other than health and viability, have also led to disquiet.

To mark the 30th birthday of IVF, the *Telegraph* will look at the breakthroughs that have changed lives – and posed dilemmas. Meanwhile, Louise, has a child of her own. Cameron, aged 18 months, was conceived naturally – an everyday miracle perhaps, but no less a miracle for that.

Multiple births: 'We were given the choice of terminating one of them, but we knew we wanted to keep all three'

The first IVF triplets were born in 1984. In recent years, the HFEA has raised concern over the relatively high incidence of multiple births conceived through IVF; the risk of death before birth or within the first week after birth is more than four times greater for twins, and almost seven times greater for triplets, than for single births. Currently, around one in four IVF pregnancies results in twins or triplets, and the HFEA is now calling for more single embryo transfers to reduce this figure to ten per cent – although clinicians are

reluctant to do so, as replacing just one embryo reduces the chance of pregnancy.

Mindy Vernon, 44, and her banker husband James, 43, live in Sevenoaks, Kent. They have triplets William, Thomas and Katherine, aged seven.

'James and I got married when I was 32 and we tried for a year and a half to have a baby, without any success. Medical tests revealed no major issues and when the doctors diagnosed unexplained infertility, we decided to go for IVF. We had three rounds of treatment at Shirley Oaks hospital, at a cost of £2,000 a cycle, which failed. By the fourth cycle we were really losing heart, so we had three embryos replaced instead of the two we'd done previously.

About 25 per cent of IVF treatments are funded by the NHS; the rest are paid for privately, costing up to £8,000 a cycle

---

'Around the time of the IVF transfer I had terrible backache, so I had acupuncture treatments for the pain. When I mentioned that I was having fertility treatment, the practitioner said she could treat that, too, by inserting the needles at other sites on my body.

'I know there's conflicting opinion about whether acupuncture increases the success of IVF. It may just have been coincidence, of course, but in my case it really did seem to work.

'When we were told we were expecting triplets, we were overjoyed that I was pregnant at all and we didn't immediately take in the significance of what it meant to be carrying three babies at once. Only later did we learn how much riskier it was for both me and the babies; we were informed that they might not all survive and were given a choice of terminating one of them. But after talking through the pros and cons, we knew we wanted to keep all three.

'I have always felt it is important to keep fit, but I was told not to exercise

and to eat as much as I could, so I stuffed myself and put on five stone. I wasn't anxious during the pregnancy, because I had faith in my body and faith in the medical staff who were looking after me. I had a really easy pregnancy, too; I wasn't badly affected by morning sickness.

'I gave up work at 22 weeks, and at 26 weeks my consultant advised me to go to hospital and stay there, so I could have complete rest and be monitored twice daily in case any problems arose. I knew I was having two boys and a girl, which the hospital had named A, B and C, and I spent my time listening to classical music and visualising them as individual little people.

'My mother was cooking for me at home every day and bringing food into the hospital, so I sat around getting fatter and feeling very special and quite serene. The babies were finally born by C-section at 34 weeks – a team of 21 doctors and nurses was involved in the delivery – and they weighed three-and-a-quarter pounds, four-and-a half pounds and five pounds. None of them had any medical problems at birth, or subsequently.

'They were allowed home after three weeks, by which time they had put on weight – and then the work really started: I breast-fed them as best I could for two months, but I didn't have much milk so they also got through 24 bottles a day.

'James and I were lucky to have lots of support from my mother, in particular, who stayed with us for a whole year, and in the first few months James's mum crossed half the country every weekend to help out.

'My mother and I did the weekday shifts and James and his mother took over at weekends so we could rest. Those early days, months and years were utterly exhausting and looking back, I can't believe we managed, but somehow we did. Having triplets is a joy, but it's also emotionally and financially draining.

'I feel ambivalent about the guidelines that only two or even just one embryo should be replaced. There's no doubt that replacing three embryos maximises a woman's chances of getting pregnant, but it's not without its medical risks and bringing up three babies is not for the fainthearted.

'Still, we were fantastically lucky with our three; we love them dearly and wouldn't swap them for the world.'

Surrogacy: 'It is about a good friend giving you the most extraordinary gift imaginable'

The first commercial surrogacy took place in Britain in 1985, when Kim Cotton, a mother of two, was paid £6,500 to carry a child conceived using her egg and the infertile woman's husband's sperm. It is now illegal for a surrogate to charge fees, but reasonable expenses may be paid to cover clothing, travel, food, time off work, etc, amounting to anything from £7,000 to £15,000.

There are two types of surrogacy. Straight surrogacy uses the egg of the surrogate and the sperm of the intended father and is usually carried out via artificial insemination at home. Host (or gestational) surrogacy requires IVF, as embryos are created using eggs and sperm from the intended mother and father and transferred into the surrogate mother.

The parents-to-be

Fiona O'Driscoll, 38, who works for the charity Save the Children, is married to Andrew, 39, a business consultant. A surrogate mother is carrying their baby, due in October.

'I have a condition called Mayer Rokitansky Kuster Hauser Syndrome (MRKH), which means I was born without a womb – although I do have ovaries – so I knew that if I wanted a family I would need to use a surrogate mother or adopt. We looked at adoption, but it's almost impossible to get a baby, and we really wanted to create one that is genetically ours.

'We got in touch with the non-profit organisation Surrogacy UK in order to make contact with a surrogate and find out more about the process. The ethos is one of friendship before surrogacy and, at the social events, we got to know another couple, Kate and Dennis, really well over a period of months. They already have two children and offered to help us.

'To be honest, my first instinct was: "Why on earth would someone offer to carry another woman's baby?" It was hard to believe anyone would do something so momentous purely out of the goodness of their own heart. But Kate is such a selfless person and she's certainly not in it for the money. It's not like the US, where you hand over tens of thousands of dollars; all we do is make sure she's not out of pocket by covering expenses like multivitamins and maternity wear, taxis and childcare.

'We were treated at the London Fertility Clinic in Harley Street; I took drugs to stimulate my egg production. These were fertilised by Andrew's sperm, and the resulting seven embryos were frozen. Two survived the thawing process and were transferred into Kate, who had taken drugs to prepare her body. Two nail-biting weeks later, Kate, Andrew and I were all together in a coffee shop in central London when the call came through that she was pregnant and we all burst into tears.

'Kate is now 28 weeks pregnant. Andrew and I – and Dennis – will all be at the birth; it's very exciting. We're so proud of what they are doing. You read horror stories about surrogacy costing a fortune or the surrogate trying to keep the baby, but the truth is, it's about a good friend giving you the most extraordinary gift imaginable.'

The surrogate mother

Kate Housely, 32, and her husband Dennis, 37, a helicopter engineer, live in Portsmouth. They have a son aged eight and a six-year-old daughter. Kate is pregnant with an IVF baby for the O'Driscolls.

'I enjoy being pregnant, but I feel very different towards this bump compared to when I was carrying my own children. I don't stroke or talk to it, I'm much more detached; I suppose it's because I've bonded with the parents, not the baby.

'It began when I read a newspaper article about surrogacy; I was intrigued, so I contacted Surrogacy UK. My main motivation was to share the great happiness that our children have brought us. At first, Dennis was baffled as to why I wanted to do this, but we went to an information day and afterwards he was every bit as keen as I was.

'Some surrogates use their own eggs; others, like me, are hosts. Before you begin, you discuss every eventuality: how many rounds of IVF you will have, what would happen if there was a problem with the foetus or if you end up being pregnant with triplets. It's important to be in agreement from the outset.

'I was previously the surrogate for another couple, but after three unsuccessful rounds of IVF the couple decided not to go any further with it. I became pregnant with Fiona and Andrew's embryo on the first IVF cycle.

'There has to be a lot of trust in any surrogacy relationship. You become a team. We've become very close and they get on brilliantly with our children, so we have no qualms about handing a baby over to them. My two children kiss my bump, but they understand that we won't be keeping the baby. I've told them that there's another mummy with a broken tummy and that I am helping her by carrying her baby.

'I don't feel as though it's my baby and there won't be any great emotional wrench when I hand him or her over; I'm really looking forward to seeing Fiona and Andrew's faces light up as

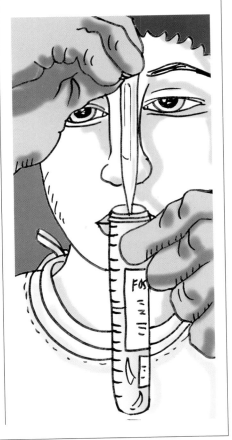

they cradle their child in their arms. For me, that's what it's all about.'

Male infertility: 'My wife and I assumed that she was to blame. I didn't expect it to be me'

The use of intracytoplasmic sperm injection (ICSI), which was introduced in 1992, has revolutionised the treatment of male infertility. It involves selecting the best sperm and injecting a single one into the cytoplasm [cell fluid] of a single egg. Male infertility accounts for 32.5 per cent of cases, and 43 per cent of all IVF treatments use this method.

Richard Clarkson, 45, who works in the music industry, is married to Anna, 39, a legal secretary. After three years of trying to conceive, they sought advice and discovered Richard had a sperm count of zero in his semen.

'I felt like I'd been punched in the solar plexus. Anna and I had both assumed the problem was on her side, and I just wasn't expecting to be the one to blame. We decided to be treated privately and went to the Assisted Reproduction and Gynaecology Centre in London, where we were told that even if there was no sperm in my ejaculate, it could be the result of a blockage or some other reason and that I could have sperm removed directly from my testes. The procedure, testicular sperm extraction (known as Tesa), involved making an incision in my scrotum and taking out tissue from which the sperm was extracted.

'I had the operation under mild sedation, and the discomfort afterwards was every bit as painful as you might imagine, but I was just so relieved the surgeon found some sperm. These were frozen and after my wife had drugs to stimulate her egg production, my sperm was used in ICSI.

'We were overjoyed when she got pregnant first time, and we now have a wonderful son who is three. At first I was mortified about how he was conceived, but these days this sort of procedure is far more common and I don't feel there's any stigma attached to any sort of IVF treatment.'

Names have been changed.

21 July 2008

UK lags behind the rest of Europe in IVF

Information from BioNews. By Antony Blackburn-Starza

Britain is languishing behind other European countries in the number of IVF cycles provided for infertile couples and Brits are three times less likely to undergo IVF than those living in Denmark and Belgium, a study reveals.

The study, led by Anders Nyboe Andersen, from Copenhagen University Hospital in Denmark, used data provided in 2006 on infertility treatment from 13 countries. The findings were presented at the annual conference of the European Society for Human Reproduction and Embryology (ESHRE) in Amsterdam last week and placed Britain 11th out of 13 countries in the number of IVF cycles undergone per million population. Denmark topped the list with 2,337 cycles per million, followed by Belgium with 2,187 cycles. In Britain, just 729 per million of the population received IVF ahead only of Germany (664) and Montenegro (408).

Commentators have interpreted the findings as illustrating the lack of funding for IVF on the National Health Service (NHS). It was reported early this year that only one in five Primary Care Trusts are providing the recommended number of IVF cycles. Clare Lewis-Jones, chief executive of Infertility Network UK, said the provision of fertility treatment in the UK was 'totally intolerable' and blamed variation across NHS Trusts in the criteria used to determine access to fertility treatment. 'We are angry that although the UK pioneered infertility treatment, we are still among the lowest providers in Europe,' she said.

Sarah Norcross, director of the Progress Educational Trust, said that there was no reason that the UK should be lagging behind the rest of Europe in its funding of infertility treatment: 'There is the political will for funding IVF, there are skilled doctors and nurses keen to treat more patients and there are women desperate for treatment,' she said. However, Dr Andersen, who led the research, said that funding was not the only factor in explaining the rankings saying that the structure in the way IVF is delivered by each country is also a determining issue.

In a separate study, also presented at the ESHRE conference, it was shown that multiple embryo transfers are commonplace in mainly Eastern European countries. The idea was raised that hundreds of British women may be travelling to such countries in the belief that multiple embryo transfers during IVF will increase their chances of conceiving. In 2006, double embryo transfers made up over 60 per cent of transfers in Bulgaria and the Ukraine. The UK's Human Fertilisation and Embryology Authority (HFEA) is promoting a single embryo transfer policy based upon safety concerns that multiple embryo transfers lead to a higher rate of multiple pregnancies, which are associated with premature birth and subsequent health problems. Mothers also face a greater health risk when carrying more than one child. Commentators believe that the lack of funding for IVF on the NHS may be persuading couples to seek treatment abroad and they could be exposing themselves to health risks in doing so.

6 July 2009

⇨ The above information is reprinted with kind permission from BioNews. Visit www.bionews.org.uk for more information.

Having children for same-sex couples

Lesbians, gay men and bisexuals are increasingly becoming parents

If you're a gay man or a lesbian woman, it doesn't mean you have to go through life without having a family of your own. The options available to potential gay and lesbian parents are wider now than ever before.

Dr Justin Varney, a public health consultant for Barking and Dagenham PCT, says: 'Gay men and lesbians are in the wonderful position where getting pregnant is a choice. It's a serious choice, but it is a choice.'

However, it's important to think through the implications of starting a family, says Dr Varney. 'There are good organisations to talk to, such as Pink Parents, or other gay parents who can tell you what having a child is like.'

Some LGB parents have children in straight relationships, which have ended. Otherwise, there are four main ways to have a child.
⇨ Donor insemination.
⇨ Co-parenting.
⇨ Adoption.
⇨ Surrogacy.

Donor insemination

This is where a man donates sperm so a woman can inseminate herself. She can be single or in a relationship.

Donor insemination can be performed at home using sperm from a friend or an anonymous donor, or at a fertility clinic using an anonymous donor.

Implications: If you decide to look for donor insemination, it's better to go to a registered clinic where the sperm is screened to ensure that it's free from sexually transmitted infections and certain genetic disorders. Fertility clinics also have support and legal advice on hand.

If you're inseminated from an anonymous donor at a fertility clinic, the 'donor' father has no legal or financial obligations to the child (although any child born after April 2005 now has the legal right to track down the biological father, so donating sperm is a significant step).

With home insemination, the male donor, whether he's a friend or anonymous, is the child's legal father and therefore has parental rights.

'It's important to find a good doctor who will talk you through all this before you make a decision,' says Dr Varney.

Speaking to your GP is a good place to start.

Co-parenting

This is typically when a lesbian and a gay man team up to have children together, although one or the other may also be straight or bisexual. The man donates the sperm and both parties share responsibility for and custody of their child.

Implications: Remember that as a co-parent you won't have sole custody of the child. It's vital to get legal advice beforehand. There are many details to be worked out, such as what role each parent will take, how financial costs will be split and the degree of involvement each will have with the child.

> 'Gay men and lesbians are in the wonderful position where getting pregnant is a choice. It's a serious choice, but it is a choice'

Adoption

Since 2002, it's been possible in England and Wales for same-sex couples to adopt a child jointly as well as being able to adopt as singletons. A bill to allow same-sex couples in Scotland the same rights is currently going through the Scottish Parliament.

Couples can apply to adopt through a local authority or an adoption agency. You don't have to live in the

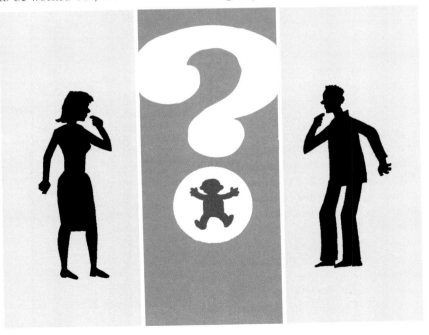

local authority you apply to.

Implications: Although most local authorities are keen to find lesbian and gay adoptive parents for children, the process can be lengthy and gruelling. Also, nearly all the children available for adoption in the UK have had traumatic backgrounds and often bring challenging behaviour as a result.

Surrogacy

Surrogacy is where another woman has a baby for a couple who can't have a child themselves. It's an option if you're a gay man, where the surrogate mother's egg can be fertilised by either you or your partner's sperm.

Implications: In reality, surrogacy is rare because it's difficult to arrange. Although it's legal in the UK,

no money other than 'reasonable expenses' can be paid to the surrogate, and there's nothing to stop her keeping the baby after it's born. It's also illegal to advertise for surrogates.
19 May 2008

⇨ Information from NHS Choices. Visit www.nhs.uk for more.

Egg and sperm donation

Information from BioCentre

A woman who provides a number of eggs (ova, oocytes) for another person or another couple who desire to have a child, is called an egg donor.

Egg donation uses the process of in vitro fertilisation. This means that the eggs are fertilised in the laboratory. Once the eggs have been obtained the role of the egg donor is completed.

IVF was first successfully performed in Britain in 1978

Egg donation may be employed in a number of clinical situations including:
⇨ The female recipient may not have any ovaries or may have ovaries that are damaged perhaps through cancer.
⇨ She may have experienced a premature menopause.
⇨ She is producing eggs which are of insufficient quality to become pregnant.
⇨ She faces the risk of passing on an inherited disorder to her child.

It is also important to note that egg donation can also be used to obtain eggs for research purposes. Human eggs that are donated to research can be used in the creation of embryos from which stem cells can be derived.

In the UK, the Human Fertilisation and Embryology Authority (HFEA) has issued a licence to the

Newcastle NHS Fertility Centre at Life to permit the practice.

Sperm donation is the name given to the process by which a man gives, or in the vast majority of cases, sells his semen to be used specifically to produce a baby. Sperm is normally donated at a sperm bank.

Recipients of donated sperm may use sperm donation for a number of reasons.
⇨ The recipient's partner may be infertile or may well carry a genetic disease.
⇨ The recipient's partner is fertile but produces low amounts of sperm or sperm of poor quality.
⇨ The recipient's partner has previously undergone a vasectomy.

⇨ In the case of a single woman, she may want to have a child but doesn't want a male partner.
⇨ Sperm donation allows a lesbian couple to have a baby.

Science and policy history
Natural procreation depends on four parental contributions, namely the father's sperm, the mother's egg, fallopian tubes which connect the mother's ovaries to her womb and where the fusion of egg and sperm take place, and the womb in which the embryo develops. Whilst this may be an oversimplification of the process, it nevertheless identifies the four main parental contributions. Should any of these four be defective in any way, it

Risk factors for IVF pregnancies

Risk	IVF pregnancy	Natural conception	Comments
Miscarriage	14-30%	15-20%	Slight increase, due to older age.
Ectopic pregnancy	1-11%	0.2-1.4%	Increase due to many factors.
Preterm delivery	24-30%	6-7%	Four-fold increase.
Small birth weight	27-32%	5-7%	Five-fold increase.
Stillbirth rate	1.2%	0.6%	Two-fold increase.
Perinatal death	2.7%	1.0%	Two-fold increase.
Congenital abnormalities	0.8-5.4%	0.8-4.5%	No significant increase.
Caesaraen section	33-58%	10-25%	Increase mainly because of multiple pregnancy and woman's age.
Multiple pregnancy			
Twins	24-31%	1.2-4.5%	
Triplets	0.5-5.2%	0.012%	Increase due to higher number of embryos transferred.
Quadruplets	0.5%	0.0001%	

Source: ivf-infertility.com

causes fertility problems. For example, infertility results if the fallopian tubes are blocked.

The sperm and egg may be fused outside the mother's body as opposed to inside it, using in vitro fertilisation (IVF). IVF was first successfully performed in Britain in 1978. Louise Brown was the first child born using the IVF technique developed by Patrick Steptoe and Robert Edwards. Since then IVF treatment has been used in a variety of contexts alongside other assisted reproductive technologies (ART).

There are a number of assisted reproductive technologies (ART):

IVF involves the use of medication to hyperstimulate the woman's ovaries to produce multiple eggs. These eggs are then extracted from the ovaries using a laparascope and mixed with sperm in a dish in the laboratory. The resulting embryos are then allowed to develop for several days in the laboratory and a small number of the embryos are subsequently implanted back into the woman's uterus.

Gamete Intrafallopian Transfer (GIFT) involves ovarian hyper-stimulation to obtain multiple eggs as with IVF. However, the eggs are then mixed with sperm and immediately placed into the women's fallopian tubes using a laparoscope. The goal of this procedure is to enable fertilisation to occur within the fallopian tubes rather than in a dish in the laboratory.

Zygote Intrafallopian Transfer (ZIFT) is rather like IVF with fertilisation of the woman's eggs taking place in the laboratory. However, unlike IVF the fertilised eggs (zygotes) are injected into the woman's fallopian tubes using a laparoscope.

Egg donation practices vary with individual cases. Some women bring their own designated donor while others rely on the services of anonymous donors. It is important to recognise that egg donation carries significant health risks to the donor mainly because of the risk of a serious adverse reaction to the medication used to induce ovarian hyperstimulation. There are a number of methods used for fertilisation, including IVF, intracytoplasmic

sperm injection (ICSI) or GIFT. The female recipient will then carry and deliver the pregnancy and keep the baby.

The first pregnancy which resulted from egg donation was in 1984.

Sperm donation involves the use of licensed donation clinics. Sperm donors are screened to meet certain requirements including age and medical history. The sperm is donated at a clinic by way of masturbation. It is then screened, washed and prepared. The sperm may then be used to inseminate a recipient woman using intrauterine insemination (IUI), or it is used to create an embryo using IVF, ICSI or other assisted reproductive treatments.

Women may decide to become egg donors for a number of reasons. Many respond to an altruistic concern for infertile couples particularly when this involves a relative or a close friend. Some assisted reproduction clinics will provide in vitro fertilisation for infertile couples at reduced cost in return for donation of eggs for use by other recipients. In the UK financial compensation for egg donors is restricted by the HFEA. However in USA and other countries it is not uncommon for women to provide eggs for significant financial compensation.

Most sperm donors are between the ages of 18-25 years and financial compensation seems to be the major motivation for donation.

Historically, sperm donation was practised under conditions of strict anonymity although physical details such as height, weight, hair colour and education were sometimes passed onto the recipient. More recently systems have been devised in some countries whereby children conceived by donor sperm may be able to obtain information about their biological father once they have reached adulthood.

Until 2002 donor anonymity still existed in the UK. However, following the case of Rose v The Secretary of Health and the HFEA, the European Human Rights Act was employed to challenge the practice of donor anonymity. This prompted the

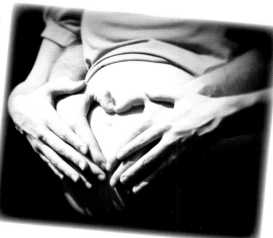
Egg and sperm donors have helped many couples to have a child

Department of Health to undertake a review of donor insemination. In 2004 the decision was taken that only sperm and egg donors who were willing to be identified at a later stage should be used, with effect from April 2005.

Since this move, there have been reports in the media of a significant decrease in donor numbers. The Government has responded by pledging further finance to help improve donor recruitment levels. Some argue for the rights of those who are infertile who undergo immense pain and distress at not being able to conceive. The loss of donor anonymity is apparently reducing the numbers of donors and therefore having an adverse effect on infertile couples. However, others argue in favour of the rights of the child to be able to know their true genetic identity. Although official policy is that children should be informed by their parents that they were conceived by donor sperm, in practice many children are never told about their biological origins. There are many stories of individuals who have experienced major psychological distress at discovering this information later in life. Some have likened it to a trap door opening up beneath them.

Ethics
ART provides couples who are unable to have children naturally, with a series of alternative options. However, as with many emerging biotechnologies, there are a number of ethical and social concerns.

Risks of egg donation

Whilst comprehensive and detailed research has not been carried out into the long-term impact of egg donation on donors, certain risks have been acknowledged.

Egg donors can suffer complications such as:
- Bleeding and trauma from the laparoscopic procedure used to obtain eggs;
- Ovarian hyperstimulation syndrome (OHSS);
- Unintended pregnancy;
- Liver failure (rare).

There is particular concern over OHSS, which arises from the use of medication to stimulate the ovaries. Whilst most cases are mild, some very severe cases have occurred. OHSS can lead to weight gain, edema, abdominal distention, pain, breathing difficulties, circulatory collapse and even death. The recognition of the real risks of egg donation has alarmed many people and brought about the convergence of groups of both pro-life and pro-choice feminists. They have voiced common concern at the way in which the health and welfare of women does not seem to be central to the planning of any biotechnological research that seeks to use the female body or tissues.

Recipients

There is a small risk that the recipient may contract an infection from donor gametes. Whilst every effort is made to reduce the risk by screening donors for a range of infections, such testing cannot provide complete protection and recent HIV infection for instance may not be detected. There are risks of undetected genetic conditions in the donor or inaccuracies in the recording and screening of the donor's medical and genetic history. All ART techniques may lead to multiple pregnancies which involve significantly increased health risks both to the mother and to the children.

The joy of being a mother

Some argue that a key advantage of egg donation is that it allows older women to become pregnant. An extreme example is 66-year-old Adriana Iliescu, who is currently the oldest women to give birth in such a way. Others argue that there are adverse consequences for the children of older women conceived by egg donation. For example, the mother may die or become too frail to care for the child, necessitating others to take on the maternal role.

Gamete market

In some countries there are signs of the development of a market for sources of egg and sperm. It is not that difficult to envisage the burgeoning of such a market as ART develops and becomes more sophisticated. There are concerns that in many countries the use of ART is not regulated in a democratically accountable way.

Commodification

ART gives greater power to potential parents to control the biological characteristics of their children. Whilst some regard this development as desirable, others argue that this implies the increasing commodification of children. It is possible that the traditional model of child bearing is shifting perspective to one of consumerism and the acquisition of a desired product.

One man: many children

Efforts have been made to try and limit the number of offspring which are created from the sperm of one donor. However, donors have the opportunity to donate at several different sperm banks and via the Internet. The DonarSiblingRegistry.com website received a posting from one man who claimed to have fathered 650 children via sperm donation.

The creation of large numbers of children from single donors raises major concerns. Firstly there is the real possibility that individuals who are unknowingly genetically related may meet and have children, a situation described as unrecognised consanguinity. As a result there is a risk of major recessive genetic disorders in subsequent offspring.

Other concerns have been raised about lack of regulation of sperm donation procedures, especially in the USA, and unrecognised genetic predispositions in donors including autism and behavioural disorders. To date little detailed research into the long-term medical and psychological outcome of children created through gamete donation has been carried out.

- The above information is reprinted with kind permission from BioCentre. Visit www.bioethics.ac.uk for more information.

© BioCentre

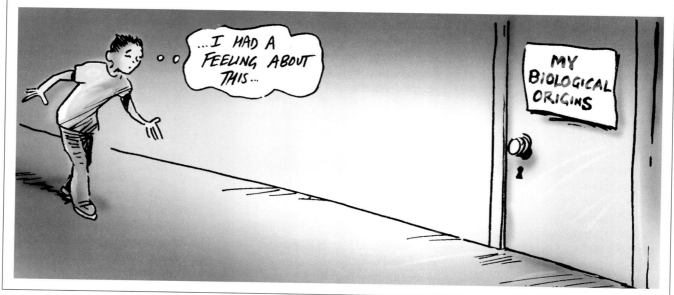

...I HAD A FEELING ABOUT THIS...

MY BIOLOGICAL ORIGINS

Addicted to surrogacy

Serena Davies reports on a Channel 4 film that examines the trend for multiple surrogate pregnancies

By Serena Davies

Tonight's Channel 4 documentary *Addicted to Surrogacy* features women who are serial surrogates. That means they've borne children for other people five, six, up to nine times, sometimes without keeping any children of their own. But this is not a sensationalist film concerned to maximise the impression that its participants are in some way unhinged. It's a sincere, moving attempt to sidestep prejudice and present surrogates as regular women who have chosen an exceptional way to help other people.

As 28-year-old Amanda, from Essex, puts it, 'I'm just helping out in the only way I can, really. Since having my own children you appreciate how lucky you are when you hear how long some people have been trying. There are a lot of people who don't deserve to have children that can have them quite easily – a lot of disgraceful mothers and fathers out there – while these couples will make good parents.'

Surrogacy has become increasingly common in Britain since the first surrogate child was born here in 1985. It has grown in popularity ever since, and Cots, one of the two main surrogacy organisations in the UK (and the company which sourced a couple for Amanda to surrogate for), recently celebrated their 600th surrogate birth. Still, the idea of a woman carrying another couple's child is not something everyone accepts easily.

To counter this, the film's director, Lucy Leveugle, says it was her priority not to place any value judgement on surrogacy. 'I think that's the point of documentary film-making,' she says. 'You're not telling the audience, you're just showing them. I didn't want to editorialise.'

Leveugle has made over 25 films focusing on sensitive human interest topics including *Child Genius*, on especially gifted children, and The *Diary of a Mail Order Bride* on Russian women who come over to marry British men (both also shown on Channel 4). She says she chose to take on the topic of surrogacy, 'because it is still such an emotive subject. It's something where we can all wonder, 'What if, one day, I'm in the position of the parents?' I wanted to know too what drives the women to become surrogates and want to do it again and again. What drives them to make such an enormous sacrifice and at what cost?'

The film focuses on four women, Jill Hawkins, Carole Horlock, Tammy Lynn and Amanda (whose surnames are not being given out). They are all paid expenses when they take on surrogacy (circa £10,000 in one instance here), but scarcely enough to suggest they're doing it for the money. Both Hawkins and Horlock are what you might call celebrity surrogates – Hawkins (44) has given away seven children, Horlock (42) holds the world record of bearing 12 surrogate children (and two of her own). Both have done press on the subject before, unlike fresh finds Tammy Lynn, an American surrogate who bears twins for a British couple in the film, and Essex-based Amanda, a first timer in the surrogate game (but with plans to take on a second) whose first surrogate pregnancy we follow.

As the film progresses and the women open up it becomes apparent that there's actually no single, easy answer to why they're taking on surrogacy.

The two married women, Carole Horlock and Tammy, seem to simply enjoy the process of being pregnant.

The cheerful Amanda, who is a single mother, seems to be partly motivated by a need for companionship. Leveugle believes Amanda became a surrogate, 'because she likes being busy, because she doesn't really have someone in her life so there's a sense of fulfilment from doing something for a couple.'

Jill Hawkins, trying – and failing – to get pregnant again at 44, seems a little desperate, perhaps the most troubled of the group. The constant surrogacy has consumed her life to the detriment of other things, notably relationships.

'Giving away babies had become too much of an emotional trauma for Jill,' says Leveugle. 'But that is true only for her.

'Surrogacy is too emotionally and personally complicated a subject matter to be able to see it in black and white. Any good documentary is about opening your eyes to a world you might not know about. I hope my film does that.'

9 March 2009

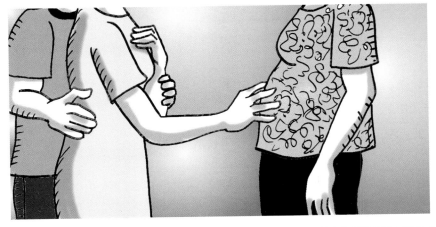

Surrogacy

The definition of surrogacy

Surrogacy is defined as follows: 'One woman (host mother or surrogate mother) carries a child for another as the result of an agreement which is made before conception that the child should be handed over after birth. The couple wishing to have the child are called the commissioning couple.' The definition is quite to the point and void of emotion. It many places, surrogacy is legal and growing in frequency.

What makes a couple choose surrogacy?

However, as with any story, there are two sides to the surrogacy tale. There is the side of the surrogate and there is also the side of the commissioning couple, particularly the mother-to-be. Many couples long for children and find, after years of fertility treatments, they are unable to conceive or carry a child of their own. Some have decided that adoption will fill their need and they bring children into their home that way. Others want to have a child that is, at least partially, biologically their own child and decide to use surrogacy to fulfill their desire.

Straight surrogacy vs. gestational surrogacy

In straight surrogacy, the host mother uses her own egg and is artificially inseminated with the sperm of the intended father. The baby then has a biological connection to the surrogate mother. Host surrogacy, also known as full or gestational surrogacy, uses the egg of the intended mother and the sperm of the intended father or an egg or sperm donor if necessary. The embryo is then implanted into the womb of the surrogate mother using IVF. There is, in this case, no biological tie between the surrogate mother and the baby. This method is the preferred way to have a surrogate birth, despite the fact that it is very costly and difficult to perform.

There are legal implications to surrogacy and there are also emotional implications to be considered before undertaking this journey. It is a very complex issue and deserves time and focus to be sure everyone is emotionally and psychologically ready to proceed. Surrogacy provides a unique option for infertile couples and it differs from adoption because it offers a couple a genetic link to their child, either from both parents or at least from one.

It involves more than 'we three'

There are more people involved in a birth by surrogacy than just the couple and the surrogate. There are families on both sides of the equation and very often other children to consider. Children need to be prepared for what is about to happen, and they need to have their questions and fears addressed. How are they going to be informed? There is also the family and friends of the commissioning couple as well as the surrogate who will have plenty of questions as well. How will these people be made aware of the decision?

Emotions and the intended mother

While the intended father will have emotions and thoughts about the surrogacy, the intended mother will have even more. She will have to be very honest about her feelings concerning the pregnancy and birth. If the surrogacy is partial, using the egg of the surrogate, how will she feel about another woman having her husband's child? Will contact be maintained with the surrogate mother? Will the child grow up knowing the circumstances of its birth? If it is a gestational surrogacy, will she be able to cope well living a pregnancy vicariously?

These and many other questions are important to consider and work through. The rewards are huge. The cost may be just as big.

⇨ The above information is reprinted with kind permission from Women's Health. Visit www.womens-health. co.uk for more information.
© Women's Health

Adoption in the UK

Information from Infertility Network UK

Throughout this article we refer to couples adopting; more and more single people and same sex couples are adopting every year. Therefore the information is applicable to anyone considering adoption.

We also refer to adopting through an Agency, this can be Local Authority (LA) or a charitable adoption agency.

Thinking about adoption

Thinking of adoption whilst still going through assisted conception treatment can seem, to many, like a simple solution – an alternative way to achieve the dream of family life. To others it can be a fall back plan should they be unsuccessful and for some, adoption is the only way forward.

However you get to the decision that adoption is right for you, it is important to spend time learning more about adoption and the impact it will have on all of your lives.

Moving on to adoption

Having decided to end treatment, or where pursuing treatment is not an option, you will still be encouraged to take some time to readjust, to have time to accept unfulfilled dreams. This can be incredibly frustrating! You are 100% committed to providing a loving family home to a child or children in need; yet have been told by your local adoption agency or Local Authority Adoption Department to go away and wait possibly six months prior to applying.

A useful tip is to use this time productively. Have a holiday, do some reading on adoption issues, speak to other adopters in different stages of the process. Attend local adoption information evenings, ask friends and family if you can spend time with their children. Subscribe to *Children Who Wait* or *Be My Parent*; two publications that detail children who are awaiting adoptive parents; this will give a feel for what children are available for adoption.

This can feel very liberating or provide clues that you are not yet ready to give up the dream of your own birth children. Listen to yourselves; if you don't feel ready then talk together or with close friends about your thoughts and feelings. This is good practice, not only for the adoption Home Study but also for coping better when you have children placed with you. When, and only when you (both) feel ready, give the agency a call.

The adoption process

The standard process for adoption is listed below and will be covered in more detail, though some agencies differ slightly:
⇨ Attendance at information evenings or initial enquiry call made to agency;
⇨ Information pack sent;
⇨ Completed application form returned;
⇨ Initial interview with applicants arranged;
⇨ Statutory checks made;
⇨ Invitation to attend prep groups
⇨ Home study begins;
⇨ Approval panel;
⇨ Children sought – the 'matching' process;
⇨ Matching panel;
⇨ Introductions;
⇨ Children placed;
⇨ Post placement support;
⇨ Adoption Order application;
⇨ Adoption Order granted;

⇨ Post adoption support;
⇨ Happily ever after...
This article will also cover:
⇨ Birth parent contact;
⇨ Legal issues;
⇨ Telling the children;
⇨ Useful resources.

Getting started

You can apply to adopt through any adoption agency. Many Local Authority agencies have formed consortiums, enabling you to undertake your home study and receive post adoption support with your local agency and have children placed from outside your region through the consortium. Where Local Authority Agencies have not formed a consortium you may be asked to apply out of your region. This is because many children are not placed in the region where they currently live.

The initial information pack ranges between informative, basic and off-putting. All packs will include an initial enquiry form, asking for basic details and often the reasons for and expectations of adoption. You may also be asked at this stage what age children you would be hoping to adopt. Agencies may have long waiting lists or not accept couples who are only interested in adopting a white baby without disabilities.

You may then be invited to either an information evening to find out more and meet the team, or an initial interview. This provides a time to ask questions about the process, to find out what children have been placed recently to give you an up to date idea of children available and time scales.

The next stage is to attend prep groups. The preparatory training introduces you to the realities of adoption. You will hear speakers, often adoptive parents who adopted through the agency and also occasionally from an adoptee. The prep groups are usually held over several weekends. The groups also aim to get you to begin to think about your own childhood and the implications from it on your adult life, in readiness for deeper exploration during the home study.

By now you will have a good idea if adoption is right for you, or not. You will be invited to either attend a second interview or complete a form detailing

if it is your intention to proceed with your application. If so, the next stage is the home study.

Continuing the process

Depending on your chosen agency, you may now have a wait until you can begin your home study. This is an assessment of the applicant's suitability to adopt and a preparation for adoptive parenthood. This will usually involve the completion of British Association for Adoption and Fostering's (BAAF) Form F3.

Information will be gathered in a series of in-depth interviews with a social worker and will include medical reports, personal references, enhanced criminal record bureau checks and other statutory checks. The home study assessment concentrates on three aspects of the applicant's lives: past experiences, current circumstances and future preparations. In addition to detailed background information on applicants, the home study will examine their understanding of the issues involved in adopting a child. LAs and all accredited agencies make no charge for the preparation of the home study report when adopting from within the UK.

When the assessment process is complete, a prospective adopter's application will be considered by the agency's adoption panel. The adoption panel is required of every adoption agency by law. The panel comprises eight or ten members and includes a mixture of professional and lay people. If approved as suitable to adopt a child, the prospective adopter's agency will look at their own files to see if they have a suitable child/children that match.

This is referred to as the matching process; it is now agreed that, wherever possible, a child should be brought up in a family of the same ethnic background as the birth parents.

Agencies also look for parents that can provide the right level of support to children with particular needs. Many agencies restrict their approved adopters' choice of children to be matched with for a set period of time, in the hope of finding them a child/children from within either their own region or another agency within their consortium.

Once that period of time has passed (maximum three months) and no child/children has been found as a suitable match, then the approved adopter/s are added to the Adoption Register operated by British Association for Adoption and Fostering (BAAF) (http://www.adoptionregister.org.uk/adoreg/default.asp).

Adopters can request not to be included on the register; they can also register themselves, three months after approval. The register contains the details of children seeking adoptive families, currently approximately four thousand. Once a match has been identified, the child's social worker is sent basic information about the prospective adoptive family. There will then be several visits from the prospective child's/children's social worker. If there is a significant possibility of the match being approved you may have the opportunity to see photographs/videos of the child/children and to speak with their current foster carer/s.

You can withdraw from the process at any time. It is important to discuss with each other and the social workers if you have any concerns at this stage. Once a match has been agreed, it has to be approved by the adoption panel.

Meeting and moving

Working together, your own and your prospective child's/children's social worker, will schedule introductions.

These arrangements will be confirmed at a planning meeting, which may be on the same day as you meet your child/children or some time beforehand.

The introductions are planned to take place over a period of days. If there is some distance between you and the child/children then the agency will fund your accommodation. There will be visits and overnight stays gradually increasing the amount of time you spend together. When all parties are comfortable, the child/children move home permanently.

Adoption leave

The Work and Families Act 2006 has made improvements to adoption leave and pay. Under this act, the Maternity and Parental Leave etc. and the Paternity and Adoption Leave (Amendment) Regulations 2006, will:

⇨ Extend maternity and adoption pay from six to nine months from April 2007, towards the goal of a year's paid leave by the end of the Parliament.

⇨ Give employed fathers a new right to up to 26 weeks Additional Paternity Leave some of which could be paid, if the mother returns to work. This will be introduced alongside the extension of adoption pay to 12 months.

An adoption does not become legal until a court makes an adoption order

Post placement support

Both yours and your child's/children's social worker will visit regularly in the early stages of placement. If you feel additional support is needed then you have a right to ask for it. Many agencies run groups as well as providing individual support, both post placement and once the adoption has been finalised.

You can gain support from Adoption UK, who help to make adoptions work, promoting loving and supportive relationships between children and their adoptive families, providing independent support, information and advice on good practice. In particular, it offers a wealth of relevant experience from generations of adoptive families.

Legalities

An adoption does not become legal until a court makes an adoption order. This transfers parental responsibility to the child's adoptive parents. Once this order is made, the birth parents no longer have any legal connection with the child.

If the adoption is contested by the birth parents the adoptive parents will be advised on seeking their own legal advice. Court costs involved are usually paid, though as in a small number of contested adoptions where the fees may be higher, the adopters may be requested to seek legal aid first. If you are in doubt, ask your social worker.

Contact with birth family

It is becoming more and more common for some form of contact to be maintained between the birth family and adopted child/children. This can be in the form of once or twice yearly letters and possibly photographs. It is, however, unusual for face-to-face contact to be maintained.

Telling

It is generally agreed that the earlier a child is aware they are adopted, the easier it is for them to grow up with that knowledge. There are now many age appropriate books and resources to help in telling your child/children that they are adopted.

Who to tell that your child is adopted remains up to you. Often some knowledge can be useful for teachers when working with different parts of the national curriculum, or if behavioural problems occur.

Your GP will have your child's/children's notes transferred following placement. You can return to the child's/children's agency at any time if further medical information is needed; though there is no guarantee new information will be available.

Resources and information

Adoption UK
46 The Green
South Bar Street
Banbury
OX16 9AB
http://www.adoptionuk.org.uk/
BAAF
Saffron House,
6-10 Kirby Street,
London,
EC1N 8TS
http://www.baaf.org.uk/
Adoption Net
http://www.adoption-net.co.uk/
Government Information on Adoption
http://www.direct.gov.uk/en/Parents/AdoptionAndFostering/index.htm

⇨ The above information is reprinted with kind permission from Infertility Network UK. Visit www.infertilitynetworkuk.com for more information on this and other related topics.

© *Infertility Network UK*

The 'test-tube baby' at 30

Deeply controversial at first, IVF has fought back ethical and religious objections to become commonplace. By Peter Singer

Louise Brown, the first person to be conceived outside a human body, turned 30 last year. The birth of a 'test-tube baby', as the headlines described in vitro fertilisation was highly controversial at the time. Leon Kass, who subsequently served as chair of President George W Bush's Council on Bioethics, argued that the risk of producing an abnormal infant was too great for an attempt at IVF ever to be justified. Some religious leaders also condemned the use of modern scientific technology to replace sexual intercourse, even when it could not lead to conception.

Since then, some three million people have been conceived by IVF, enabling otherwise infertile couples to have the child they longed for. The risk of having an abnormal child through IVF has turned out to be no greater than when parents of a similar age conceive through sexual intercourse. However, because many IVF practitioners transfer two or three embryos at a time to improve the odds of a pregnancy occurring, twins and higher multiple births are more common, and carry some additional risk.

The Catholic church has not moved away from its opposition to IVF. In a recently released instruction, *Dignitas Personae*, the Church's Congregation for the Doctrine of the Faith objects to IVF on several grounds, including the fact that many embryos are created in the process, and few survive. This outcome is not, however, very different from natural conception, for the majority of embryos conceived by sexual intercourse also fail to implant in the uterine wall, with the woman often not even knowing that she was ever 'pregnant'.

In addition, the Vatican objects to the fact that conception is the result of a 'technical action' rather than 'a specific act of the conjugal union'. But while any couple would prefer to conceive a child without the intervention of doctors, that option is not available for infertile couples. In those circumstances, it is harsh to say to a couple that they cannot have their own genetic child at all.

Some three million people have been conceived by IVF

It also appears contrary to the broad thrust of the church's teaching about marriage and the family as the appropriate context for rearing children. *Dignitas Personae* says that new human life should be 'generated through an act which expresses the reciprocal love between a man and a woman'. But if by that the church is referring to sexual intercourse, then it surely has an unduly narrow view of what kinds of acts can express reciprocal love between a man and a woman. Taking the several inconvenient and sometimes unpleasant steps required to have a child together by means of IVF can be, and often is, the result of a much more deliberate and reciprocally loving act than sexual intercourse.

A better objection to IVF is that in a world with millions of orphaned or unwanted children, adoption is a more ethical way of having a child. If that is the argument, however, why should we single out couples who use IVF? Why not, for example, criticise Jim Bob and Michelle Duggar, the Arkansas couple who recently had their 18th child? Yet Michelle Duggar was named 'Young Mother of the Year' in Arkansas in 2004, when she had already given birth to 14 children. I haven't noticed the Vatican telling them that they should be adopting instead of conceiving so many children.

Religious opposition notwithstanding, the use of IVF by infertile couples of normal reproductive age has been widely accepted around the world, and rightly so. But in countries where the church's influence remains strong, IVF's opponents are fighting back. In Poland, for example, proposed new legislation would drastically restrict its availability.

Elsewhere, the ethical debate is not about IVF itself, but the limits of its use. Last November, Rajo Devi, a 70-year-old Indian woman, became the world's oldest mother, thanks to IVF. She and her 72-year-old husband have, she says, longed for a child through 55 years of marriage. Her husband's sperm appears to have been used, but news reports are unclear about the source of the egg.

Some will find it grotesque to become a mother at an age when most women are grandmothers, but the more significant question is what kind of care such children will have if their parents die or become incapable of rearing them. Like many people in rural India, Devi lives in an extended family with other relatives, so she is confident that there would be others to bring up her child if necessary.

But, as this example suggests, the impact of parental age on a child's welfare will vary from one culture to another. Becoming a mother at 70 is more acceptable for someone living in a joint family than it would be for western couples living in their own home without close relatives or friends nearby.

14 January 2009
© *Guardian News & Media Ltd 2009*

Fertility tourism

Survey finds three-quarters of fertility patients would consider going abroad for treatment

An online survey of more than 300 fertility patients carried out for National Infertility Day has found that 76% would consider travelling overseas for their treatment. 30 years after the first IVF baby was born in the UK, the cost of fertility treatment here plus long waiting lists have proved the decisive factor when it comes to patients choosing to go abroad instead.

88% of those who had had treatment abroad were happy with the service they received, and that's not just down to the cost and shorter waiting lists

There's been growing interest in 'fertility tourism', but this survey carried out by Infertility Network UK for this year's National Infertility Day taking place on 19 July is the first detailed research into the subject. It shows that 88% of those who had had treatment abroad were happy with the service they received, and that's

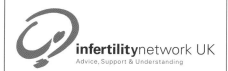

infertitynetwork UK
Advice, Support & Understanding

not just down to the cost and shorter waiting lists. High success rates, the attitude of staff, the atmosphere of clinics and the facilities have all impressed patients from the UK when they travel for treatment.

Shortages of donor eggs and sperm in the UK have been sending many overseas, but the survey results suggest that others who don't need to use donor eggs or sperm are now joining the fertility exodus.

Of the 24% of the patients surveyed who said they wouldn't consider going abroad most were concerned about standards in clinics abroad, lack of regulation and language problems.

Clare Brown, Chief Executive of Infertility Network UK said: 'If the NHS funded three full cycles of treatment as recommended by the National Institute for Health and Clinical Excellence (NICE), many couples would not be forced to consider going abroad for treatment. It is absolutely vital that anyone

considering travelling abroad should do some thorough research beforehand as the rules and regulations abroad can be totally different from those in the UK. I do hope though that clinics in the UK take into account the findings of this survey and learn from the good experiences many couples have had at clinics abroad.'

The results of the survey will be presented at a conference for patients as part of National Infertility Day on 19 July in central London. National Infertility Day is open to anyone with an interest in fertility, and will be attended by a wide range of speakers including IVF pioneer, Professor Robert Edwards and ICSI (Intracytoplasmic sperm injection) pioneer Andre Van Steirteghem from Brussels.

Key findings

⇨ 339 people responded to the survey, and 76% of them would consider travelling abroad for treatment.

⇨ The main attractions of overseas fertility clinics were short waiting times and the cost of treatment (70% of those who said they'd consider treatment abroad listed these as attractions). These were closely followed by success rates (61%) and the availability of donor eggs and sperm (54%).

⇨ The majority of those who'd had treatment abroad had been happy with the experience (88%), and for those who had problems, most of these (47%) were due to difficulties with language and communications and (37%) lack of regulation.

15 July 2008

⇨ The above information is reprinted with kind permission from Infertility Network UK. Visit www.infertilitynetworkuk.com for more information.

© *Infertility Network UK*

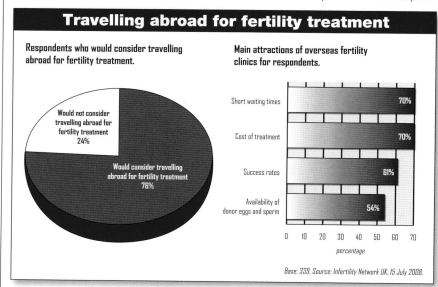

Travelling abroad for fertility treatment

Respondents who would consider travelling abroad for fertility treatment.

- Would not consider travelling abroad for fertility treatment 24%
- Would consider travelling abroad for fertility treatment 76%

Main attractions of overseas fertility clinics for respondents.

	percentage
Short waiting times	70%
Cost of treatment	70%
Success rates	61%
Availability of donor eggs and sperm	54%

0 10 20 30 40 50 60 70

Base: 339. Source: Infertility Network UK, 15 July 2008.

Is 66 too old to have a baby?

Elizabeth Adeney, a wealthy divorcee from Suffolk, has revealed she is eight months pregnant with her first child, conceived via IVF treatment in Ukraine. Where's the harm in that?

By Laura Donnelly and Graham Stack

Last summer, days before the christening of her baby daughter Freya was due, new mother Susan Tollefsen was rushed to hospital. Celebrations were put on hold: doctors discovered a burst ulcer that required surgery.

It was one of four major operations Mrs Tollefsen was to undergo in the first four months of motherhood, including one to replace a knee joint. If she had wished to forget her status as Britain's oldest first-time mother at the age of 57, her sudden frailty was a brutal reminder.

'It made me realise how susceptible you are if your health goes,' she says. 'All the fears I had about being an older mum had dimmed because everything was going so well. It did make me rethink. I wished I wasn't this old.'

Most of the time, she brushes away such thoughts, along with those that come to mind when strangers mistake her for Freya's grandmother or other mothers attack her decision to seek fertility treatment at the age of 56. 'Yes, I wish I was 20 or 30 years younger, but I am so over the moon that I have a child,' she says.

Forced by critics to defend her decision to conceive a child by a donor egg and sperm at a Russian fertility clinic in 2007, she explains how she met her husband Nick, 46, late in life, after nursing her elderly mother for much of her adulthood. Not everyone is sympathetic; after a trip to her local mother and baby clinic in Essex, Mrs Tollefsen left in tears.

Nevertheless, for the special needs teacher, who is about to take early retirement to spend more time with her daughter, the very existence of her one year old makes it all worthwhile. She recalls: 'When I saw first saw Freya, I said I've waited for you for so long – but my goodness you were worth the wait.'

Mrs Tollefson is not the oldest woman in the UK to have a child. In a fertility race that has horrified many commentators, that record was set three years ago, when Patricia Rashbrook, 62, from Sussex, gave birth to a son using an egg from a donor in Russia. Dr Rashbrook attracted particular opprobrium because although the child was her husband's first, she already had three grown-up children.

'I think the idea of setting out knowing that a child is quite likely not to have a parent by their 18th birthday is alarming'

Yesterday, another British woman looked set to smash through both records. At 66, Elizabeth Adeney, a wealthy divorcee from Suffolk, is eight months pregnant with her first child, conceived via IVF treatment in Ukraine.

All three women travelled abroad for treatment because most British clinics will not offer services to women above the age of 50.

Mrs Adeney, the managing director of a textiles firm in Mildenhall, is said to have been 'desperate' for a baby, in perfect health and thrilled to discover that she had fallen pregnant, her friends said.

Not everyone saw it that way. The news immediately reopened a fierce debate about whether medical advances have gone beyond what is best for society – and, above all, best for children.

The Suffolk woman will be 79 by the time her child reaches its teens. Yesterday, chatrooms and dinner parties were alive with debate about the case.

On Mumsnet, the parenting website, many mothers expressed sympathy for others who had found a chance of motherhood late in life. Many of the women who use the site to share their experiences of motherhood have become parents of advanced years, and there are even specific discussion groups for women in their forties undergoing fertility treatment. Yet the vast majority described the need for a 'cut-off point', with several accusing the likes of Mrs Adeney of an 'act of breathtaking selfishness'.

But on Radio 4 last week, as broadcaster John Humphreys pointed out that Mrs Adeney would be in her eighties by the time her child reached University, fertility expert Dr Gillian Lockwood gently highlighted a double standard in the way older parents are

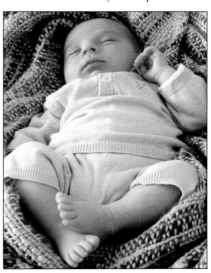

treated, depending on their gender. Humphreys, now 66, hit the headlines a decade ago when he announced he was to have a third child at the ripe old age of 56.

As Dr Lockwood, vice president of the Royal College of Obstetricians and Gynaecologists ethics committee, wryly noted, when Humphreys announced the news 'it was cigars all round', much as it was when fellow BBC broadcaster Jonathan Dimbleby later had a child at the age of 64.

Humphreys took the dig in good humour, while acknowledging Dr Lockwood's point, that life expectancy for women outstrips that of men.

Dr Lockwood told the *Sunday Telegraph*: 'It's a brute biological fact that life expectancy has almost doubled in the past century, whereas reproductive expectancy is almost unchanged.'

Most British clinics will not offer services to women above the age of 50

Today, a woman of 65 has a life expectancy of 85, while the average man lives to 82. Both figures are predicted to continue rising.

Screening for women undergoing fertility treatment means those who are allowed to proceed are likely to be healthier than average, she adds. And because IVF treatments for older women rely on donated eggs taken from younger women, almost all of the dangers to the child associated with older motherhood – such as increased risks of Down's syndrome and other foetal abnormalities – are not present. Risks to the mother, such as pre-eclampsia, a condition linked to high blood pressure, can be minimised if correctly monitored.

Dr Lockwood says: 'As long as a woman is fit and healthy and doesn't have an underlying health problem, like diabetes or blood pressure, the risk is not that great.'

She believes the safety of childbirth for older women is one of the least difficult assessments to make. The fundamental problem is examining what she describes as 'the psychological aspect' of each case.

'If it is a single woman seeking motherhood in their forties, I would be asking why now, why is it that they aren't content to be aunts or godmothers? You have to be careful that it hasn't become too much of a fixation, and you have to check that someone isn't seeking a nurse or companion, that the needs of the child are coming first.'

While the NHS will only provide fertility treatment up to the age of 40, Dr Lockwood does not believe age alone should be used as 'a cut-off point'.

'I don't think it's acceptable just to say that someone who would be a good mother at 49 and a half, but they are unacceptable at 50.'

Many private clinics do not have an explicit cut-off point. But with a long queue for donor eggs, few will provide them to women over the age of 50 – in many cases because those women donating eggs specify that they do not want them to go to post-menopausal women, she says.

In other cases, women whose biological clock has already run out are not prepared to sit on a waiting list for years to see if they can get lucky. As a result, many become 'fertility tourists' visiting clinics abroad, with Ukraine, a former Soviet state, particularly popular.

The use of clinics abroad, where women may not be properly monitored throughout both treatment and pregnancy, concerns Dr Lockwood and other fertility experts in the UK – and far more than the fact of late motherhood.

While the Isida fertility clinic in Kiev, one of Ukraine's leading centres, refused to confirm rumours that its doctors treated Elizabeth Adeney, its marketing manager Pavel Oltarzhevsky told the *Sunday Telegraph* that it was rare for women of Adeney's age to seek treatment. Shockingly, he said the only consideration its doctors made was whether the woman was willing; factors such as age, and even the health of the patient were disregarded.

'Age is no consideration,' said Mr Oltarzhevsky. 'Willingness is the only thing that counts. We would even treat an 80 year old. If she really wants it, then she can really get it.'

Asked what health factors the doctors would take into account, he replied: 'Successful IVF is our goal. Then the patients return to their home countries for pregnancy and birth, and we usually never hear from them again. The only thing the IVF department deals with is IVF.'

He underlined his point: 'There is no feedback or follow-up procedure. We have no way of knowing what happens later to them or their babies. We do not call them and they do not, as a rule, call us.'

His frank admissions underline concerns expressed by British fertility experts. Dr Allan Pacey, secretary of the British Fertility Society, believes the limits to fertility treatment within the UK are set correctly at around the age of 50 – and that more should be done to discourage 'fertility tourism', especially those cases where desperate women 'find a clinic on the Internet, a cheap flight and go'.

'In those cases, they can end up with no British clinic knowing anything of the reputation of the clinic abroad, and no one monitoring their health once they return to this country. That is one of the things that concerns me most. We have seen cases in which it has turned out that they have been treated by people who are not even qualified medics.'

Even with lengthening life expectancy, Dr Pacey believes that women seeking motherhood in their sixties are taking too large a gamble. 'People will say that you can't predict when a parent will die: some children are orphaned in tragic accidents. That is true, but I think the idea of setting out knowing that a child is quite likely not to have a parent by their 18th birthday is alarming.'

He adds: 'Most people feel uncomfortable about the idea of providing fertility treatment to women beyond the natural menopause. In some ways, setting a cut-off point of 50 is arbitrary. But when you combine the welfare of the child, the health of the mother, and, indeed, the "yuk" factor of society, I think that is a reasonable place to end up.'
16 May 2009

Health problems for IVF twins

Twins born after fertility treatment have a higher risk of problems at birth and in the first three years of life. Second study finds reassuring evidence on the outcome of children born after embryo freezing

Twins born as a result of assisted reproductive technology (ART) are more likely to be admitted to neonatal intensive care and to be hospitalised in their first three years of life than spontaneously conceived twins, according to new research published online today (Wednesday 20 May) in Europe's leading reproductive medicine journal *Human Reproduction*[1].

It is known already that ART twins are at higher risk of problems such as low birth weight and premature delivery than singletons around the time of their birth, but, to a large extent, these risks exist as part of the problems associated with multiple births in general. Up to now there has been conflicting evidence about whether assisted reproduction itself is responsible for adding to the number of problems seen in ART twins.

To answer this question, researchers in Australia and the UK looked at perinatal outcomes and hospital admissions for all twin children born in Western Australia between 1994 and 2000, whether as a result of ART or spontaneous conception.

Twins that arise as a result of ART usually do so because two (or sometimes more) separate embryos are implanted in the woman's womb. They are non-identical and each has its own placenta. However, twins that arise as a result of spontaneous conception can either be non-identical because two eggs have been fertilised at the same time, or identical because one fertilised egg has divided to make two embryos. Identical twins share a placenta in about two-thirds of all cases, and this is associated with an increased risk of death and other complications. In order to ensure that, as far as possible,

they were comparing like for like, the researchers matched the ART twins with spontaneously conceived, non-identical twins of different sexes (referred to in the study as 'unlike sex spontaneously conceived twins', or 'ULS SC twins').

Embryos that had been frozen shortly after they started to divide had a better, or at least as good, obstetric outcome as children born from fresh cycles of IVF

Michèle Hansen, a researcher and PhD student at the Telethon Institute for Child Health Research in Western Australia, said: 'We found that twins conceived following ART treatment had a greater risk of adverse perinatal outcome, including preterm birth, low birthweight and death, compared

with spontaneously conceived twins of unlike sex. ART twins had more than double the risk of perinatal death compared to ULS SC twins, although the risk was similar to that of all SC twins, including identical twins.

'ART twins stayed longer in hospital than ULS SC twins at the time of their birth: an average of 12 days compared with eight days. ART twins were four times more likely to be admitted to neo-natal intensive care than ULS SC twins, and were more likely to be admitted to hospital during the first three years of their life. After adjusting for confounding factors such as year of birth, maternal age, parity and so on, ART twins still had a nearly two-thirds higher risk of being admitted to neo-natal intensive care, and a higher risk of being admitted to hospital in their first three years of life, although this was only statistically significant in their second year, when their risk was nearly two-thirds higher.'

Ms Hansen continued: 'Couples undergoing fertility treatment should be aware that, in addition to the known

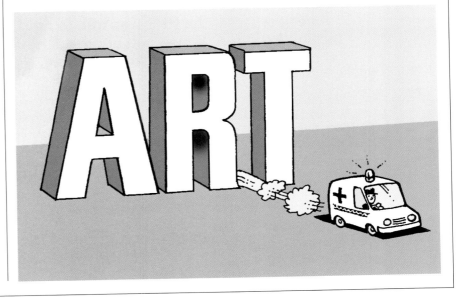

increased perinatal risks associated with a twin birth, ART twins are more likely than spontaneously conceived twins to be admitted to neonatal intensive care and to be hospitalised in their first three years of life.

'We don't know the reason for the increased risks of adverse perinatal outcome and hospitalisation and preliminary analysis of specific diagnoses does not provide any answers. The underlying causes of parental infertility and/or components of the ART procedure may be increasing the risks of adverse outcome, and increased concern about children born after a long period of infertility may also be contributing to their increased risk of hospitalisation. Estimates of the cost of an ART twin delivery should take into account these increased risks, and, in order to reduce the problems associated with twin births, clinicians and couples should consider the benefits of opting for single embryo transfer.'

A second study, also published online today in *Human Reproduction*, provides reassuring evidence on the outcome of children born after embryos were frozen and stored, before being thawed and transferred to the womb[2]. The results are good news as an increasing number of children, estimated to be 25% of ART

babies worldwide, are now born after freezing or vitrification (a process similar to freezing that prevents the formation of ice crystals).

The study, led by Dr Ulla-Britt Wennerholm, an obstetrician at the Institute for Clinical Sciences, Sahlgrenska Academy (Goteborg, Sweden), reviewed the evidence from 21 controlled studies that reported on prenatal or child outcomes after freezing or vitrification.

She found that embryos that had been frozen shortly after they started to divide (early stage cleavage embryos) had a better, or at least as good, obstetric outcome (measured as preterm birth and low birth weight) as children born from fresh cycles of IVF (in vitro fertilisation) or ICSI (intracytoplasmic sperm injection). There were comparable malformation rates between the fresh and frozen cycles. There were limited data available for freezing of blastocysts (embryos that have developed for about five days) and for vitrification of early cleavage stage embryos, blastocysts and eggs.

'Slow freezing of embryos has been used for 25 years and data concerning infant outcome seem reassuring with even higher birthweights and lower rates of preterm and low birthweights than children born

after fresh IVF/ICSI. For the newly introduced technique of vitrification of blastocysts and oocytes, very limited data have been reported on obstetric and neonatal outcomes. This emphasises the urgent need for properly controlled follow-up studies of neonatal outcomes and a careful assessment of evidence currently available before these techniques are added to daily routines. In addition, long-term follow-up studies are needed for all cryopreservation techniques,' concluded Dr Wennerholm.

References

1 Twins born following assisted reproductive technology: perinatal outcomes and admissions to hospital. *Human Reproduction*. doi:10.1093/humrep/dep173

2 Children born after cryopreservation of embryos or oocytes: a systematic review of outcome data. *Human Reproduction*. doi:10.1093/humrep/dep125

20 May 2009

⇨ The above information is reprinted with kind permission from the European Society of Human Reproduction and Embryology. Visit www.eshre.com for more.

© European Society of Human Reproduction and Embryology

No end to IVF 'postcode lottery'

Five years after the NHS was told to fund three cycles of fertility treatment for women under 40, new research shows access to IVF is still a postcode lottery. Roz Upton reports

Only one in five Primary Care Trusts (PCTs) questioned by Conservative MP Grant Shapps are providing the allocated number of cycles.

The National Institute for Clinical Excellence (Nice) guidelines on age are also being ignored with women being told they are too old for treatment in one part of the country and too young in another.

Two PCTs have refused women any

IVF in the previous two years while one in eight PCTs is failing to comply with guidelines on a woman's age. In the east midlands, every trust offers one full cycle of treatment, but in the south east, 41 per cent do not offer IVF to any woman aged 23 to 39, as set out in the guidance.

Overall, 54 per cent of trusts exclude couples from IVF if one partner has a child from a previous relationship. In the east midlands,

no PCT would offer treatment to couples in which one partner already has a child but 70 per cent would in the north east.

Almost half of all trusts said they wanted couples to have been in a relationship for more than three years, but others said one or two years while some merely asked that the relationship was 'stable'.

The study, based on freedom of information requests from Tory MP

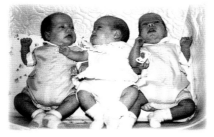

The NHS wants to cut the number of multiple births arising as a result of IVF

Grant Shapps, was based on an 80 per cent response rate from PCTs in England.

Experts have warned that the drive to cut the number of multiple births is also being hampered by the lack of access to free IVF. Couples who have the chance of only one cycle on the NHS may wish to have more than one embryo transferred, they said.

The Nice guidance also said PCTs should allow frozen embryos to be transferred as part of one complete IVF cycle on the NHS. But very few PCTs offer this.

Experts have warned that the drive to cut the number of multiple births is also being hampered by the lack of access to free IVF

Mr Shapps said: 'IVF remains a postcode lottery in this country.'

He added: 'Budgets are tight and the NHS must set its priorities, but it is wrong to raise expectations in couples who are desperate to start a family only for them to find out later that they won't get the real help they expected.'

A spokesman for the Department of Health said: 'Our survey of every PCT in England shows the NHS is making good progress in implementing Nice guidelines and in providing fair and consistent access to IVF.'
6 August 2009

⇨ The above information is re-printed with kind permission from Channel 4. Visit www.channel4.com for more information.

© Channel 4

Winston: egg freezing is 'expensive confidence trick'

Information from BioNews. By Benjamin Jones

Lord Winston, emeritus Professor of Fertility Studies at Imperial College London and pioneer of IVF, has criticised fertility clinics for over-hyping egg freezing services. In an interview with the *Daily Mail* newspaper he accuses providers of creating false optimism in the effectiveness of the procedure, particularly where signing up patients for purely 'social' reasons. Before use of egg freezing grows further he calls for more research into both the effects of egg freezing on the ability to later conceive and into the long-term health implications for those born from frozen eggs.

The comments come in response to calls, made at this week's European Society for Human Reproduction and Embryology (ESHRE) annual conference, for greater availability of egg freezing as an option for women who are postponing pregnancy until later in their lives. Lord Winston's comments partially mirror a joint statement made in February by the UK's Royal College of Obstetricians and Gynaecologists and the British Fertility Society (BFS) which also called for women not to freeze eggs for social reasons.

Lord Winston noted that the production of six to ten eggs for freezing involves both the risk of ovarian hyperstimulation syndrome for the woman and an increased likelihood of chromosome defects in the eggs produced. Producing such a quantity of eggs he sees as dangerous yet also inadequate to ensure a viable embryo is produced. The BFS has stated that the average chance of success for any individual frozen egg is six per cent and only four children have been born from frozen eggs in the UK to date.

Additionally, the lack of data on the long-term health effects – the first children conceived with frozen eggs are only now five – is provided as reason enough for adopting a cautious approach towards increasing availability of egg freezing and makes encouraging those without a pressing need (such as impending cancer treatment) all the more dubious. Lord Winston states, in unequivocal terms, 'in my view it is irresponsible [for clinics] to egg freeze until long-term animal research has been done'. The most detailed research to date is due to be published next month.

Describing the procedure as a 'quick fix', Lord Winston sees the best path forward for prolonging the ability to have a child, for social reasons, is to attempt to develop better means of postponing the menopause. Though the procedure can be justified for those with serious medical conditions it is not to be encouraged as a means of delaying motherhood. The provision of egg freezing for social reasons, available for between £2,500 and £5,000 at 45 clinics in the UK, is in his view simply an 'undesirable commercial activity' and should not be encouraged.
3 July 2009

⇨ The above information is reprinted with kind permission from BioNews. Visit www.bionews.org.uk for more information.

© BioNews

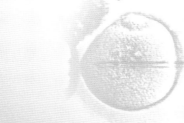

The donor crisis

Childless couples denied as anonymity loss scares egg and sperm donors

By Mark Henderson, Science Editor

The removal of anonymity from sperm and egg donors has provoked a crisis in fertility treatment that is denying couples the chance to try for a baby.

Infertility therapy with donated sperm has collapsed to the lowest levels since records began, according to the first official figures, seen by The Times, since the Government banned anonymous donation in 2005.

The number of women treated with donated sperm fell by about 20 per cent, from 2,727 in 2005 to 2,107 in 2006, the first full year after the change. The number of donor insemination treatment cycles fell by 30 per cent over the same period.

Egg donation is also in serious decline: the number of treatments using 'shared' eggs, offered by women in return for a discount on IVF, fell by 40 per cent between 2004 and 2006.

The figures demolish claims by ministers and the Human Fertilisation and Embryology Authority (HFEA) that sperm donation has improved since anonymity was ended. Last year Shirley Harrison, then the chairwoman of the authority, said it was 'a myth' that there had been problems.

Although the number of sperm donors has risen slightly, many will be friends and relatives who donate for a couple's exclusive use. Fewer donors are contributing to sperm banks, from which the donation can be used by up to ten women. The result is that although more donors have been registered, the shortage of sperm is becoming more acute.

The law, which took effect on 1 April 2005, gives donor-conceived children the right to trace their biological parents when they reach 18. The Government said that children's rights to discover their genetic origins outweighed donors' right to privacy. Many doctors, however, predicted that this would worsen an existing shortage of sperm and eggs, because donors would worry about being approached later in life.

Most clinics now have waiting lists of at least two years for sperm, and a similar trend is affecting egg donation. Although altruistic donation, which is usually done by sisters or friends for a patient's exclusive use, has remained static, the egg-sharing schemes that help couples without a known donor are in trouble. Shared eggs were used in only 680 fertility procedures in 2006, compared with 1,142 in 2004, the last year before the law was changed.

Infertility therapy with donated sperm has collapsed to the lowest levels since records began

MPs and fertility doctors say the figures show that the end of anonymity has denied treatment to thousands of infertile men and women.

Evan Harris, the Liberal Democrat science spokesman, said: 'The Government and the HFEA have been saying everything is fine, but it isn't. There was no good reason for removing anonymity, which has led to a catastrophic drop in the number of patients treated by donor insemination.

'There was always a huge risk that this would happen, diminishing the capacity of both the NHS and private clinics to treat infertility. There are probably now thousands of untreated couples who may be forced abroad, or into the unregulated sector.'

Gillian Lockwood, medical director of Midland Fertility Services, said her clinic had performed 83 treatment cycles with donated sperm last year, compared with 221 in 2004.

'The picture at the coal face is bleak,' she said. 'A significant number of patients are now being turned into fertility tourists, who are going abroad for donor treatment.'

A spokesman for the Department of Health confirmed that the number of egg donors had fallen. 'We are therefore preparing a regional egg donor recruitment campaign which will be launched in stages from July,' he said.

A spokeswoman for the HFEA said: 'The HFEA supports the efforts of clinics actively recruiting donors.'

Pip Morris, of the National Gamete Donation Trust, said: 'We've never had enough donors. It's nothing to do with the law, it's a lack of awareness.'

26 June 2008

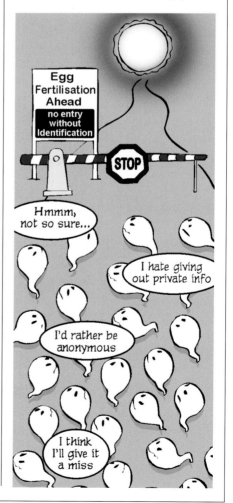

Sperm donors are curious too

Information from the Economic and Social Research Council

The popular image of sperm donors as being desperate to avoid any contact with their donor offspring is false. New research from Edinburgh University shows men who donated semen anonymously in the past are not necessarily comfortable with being unaware of the outcome of their donations. Many hope that life has turned out well for offspring created as a result of their donations. Some donors, it appears, hope that they may be traced by donor offspring and would then treat them as members of their family.

> **Some donors, it appears, hope that they may be traced by donor offspring and would then treat them as members of their family**

Research was carried out at the ESRC Innogen Centre at Edinburgh University, as part of a PhD thesis, exploring what it meant to men who donated semen between the 1960s and early 1980s, how they are experiencing the culture of secrecy so characteristic of gamete donation, and whether their views about having donated have changed.

Contrary to expectations, every donor had told at least one person in their social network that they had donated semen. This was usually their wife but also included children, colleagues, friends and other relatives. However, the identity of donors remains hidden from offspring unless both parties have registered with UK Donorlink, a voluntary contact register run by After Adoption Yorkshire. In addition, many clinic

esrc | **society today**

records were destroyed prior to 1990 when donor insemination became subject to regulation by the Human Fertilisation and Embryology Act.

None of the donors had been told that their donations resulted in the birth of healthy babies but most donors presume that this is the case, especially men who are aware that a clinic's policy was to limit to five the number of children conceived with the help of each donor. A few donors have chosen to assume that no children resulted, and for them any discussion about a sense of connection to donor offspring is theoretical. This is also the case for donors who know that their semen was mixed with the semen of other donors or with the husbands of the recipients before insemination, as a way of ensuring that paternity could not be attributed to a particular donor. This practice was common in some clinics until it was deemed too risky due to the increasing emphasis on the importance of the traceability of human tissues and gametes.

When donors think that donor offspring exist, they often admit to curiosity about what these individuals look like, especially whether they might resemble the donor, his children, or his siblings and cousins. A genetic connection between a donor and his donor-conceived children is thought to imply that the two individuals will look alike or at least share some similar features and dispositions.

The idea of possible contact with donor offspring is influenced by perceptions and experiences of what it means to be a parent. Donors who have personal or professional knowledge of adoption, fostering or step-parenting are likely to understand that donor-conceived people might want to meet them, or at least have access to personal information about them. These and other donors recognise that different kinds of relatives, including donors, are able to play a non-interfering role in the lives of donor offspring and that they are not necessarily the door-stepping fortune hunters often suggested in the media.

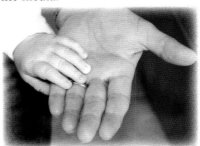

A significant legacy of the historical development of donor insemination in the UK, however, is that legislation did not introduce protection for donors from inheritance claims from donor offspring. Although there is no evidence that such claims will be made, the thought of it is a worry for some donors' wives. The Human Fertilisation and Embryology Bill soon to be introduced in the House of Commons would provide an opportunity to rectify this problem. *March 2008*

⇨ The above information is taken from the Economic and Social Research Council publication *The Edge*, Issue 27, and is reprinted with permission. Visit www.esrc.ac.uk for more information.
© Economic and Social Research Council

Donors creating new forms of extended families

New family connections are formed when parents of donor-conceived children seek out the donors and their other children. Findings of new study have wider implications for policy in this area

Parents who have conceived children with the help of sperm or egg donors and then try to find the donors and also other children conceived with the donors' help, often end up creating new forms of extended families, according to research published today (Tuesday 24 February).

The study in Europe's leading reproductive medicine journal *Human Reproduction*,[1] found that parents set out to find their children's donor and other donor siblings through feelings of curiosity and a desire to enhance their children's sense of identity, and without expecting any very close contact. However, once they had identified the donor and their children's donor siblings, they not only found the experiences of contacting and meeting the donor siblings very positive, but in many cases formed close and continuing bonds.

Dr Tabitha Freeman, a research associate at the Centre for Family Research, University of Cambridge (UK), said: 'Our most important finding is that the practice of donor conception is creating new family forms. These family forms are based on genetic links between families with children conceived by the same donor, as well as between donor-conceived children's families and their donors' families. Contrary to what might be expected, this research has found that contact between these new family forms can be a very positive experience for those involved. One very striking finding is that family members in this sample formed close links based on notions of family and kinship; for example, the mothers experienced maternal feelings towards their children's donor siblings.

'In addition, it is very interesting that this process is being driven by parents of donor-conceived children who, whilst having conceived using anonymously donated sperm, regard it as important for their children to have access to information about their genetic relations.'

An overwhelming majority of parents reported positive experiences of contacting and meeting their child's donor siblings and donor

---

Dr Freeman and colleagues recruited 791 parents via the Donor Sibling Registry, a US-based international registry that facilitates contact between donor conception families who share the same donor. The parents completed an online questionnaire and data were collected on their reasons for searching for their child's donor siblings and/or the donor, the outcome of these searches and the parents' and children's experiences of any resulting contact.

The parents consisted of 39% lone mothers, 35% lesbian couples and 21% heterosexual couples. In this study, 91% (717) of parents lived in the United States, 5% (37) in Canada and 1% (8) in the UK; other countries of residence included Austria, Germany, Ireland, Spain, Sweden, Australia, New Zealand and Israel. Some parents had discovered large numbers of donor siblings; 11% (55) of parents who had found their child's donor siblings had found ten or more, with one parent finding as many as 55. An overwhelming majority of parents reported positive experiences of contacting and meeting their child's donor siblings and donor. They frequently described feeling excited and happy on their child's behalf when they found donor siblings, and viewed the addition of such relationships to their children's lives as 'enriching', 'wonderful' and 'fun'.

Dr Freeman said the findings have wider implications for research and policy, particularly as an increasing number of countries have removed the right to donor anonymity.

In the paper, the authors write: 'The finding that parents placed more importance on tracing and establishing contact with their child's donor siblings than their child's donor has important implications for research and policy in this field. In particular, it is crucial that donor siblings are incorporated into discussions about the regulation of gamete donation, with a key consideration being the number of donor offspring to be conceived using any one donor. The potential for parents and children to form relationships with members of families who share the same donor is a significant consequence of the removal of donor anonymity that has yet to receive adequate attention. This study shows that, while the donor sibling relationship lies at the centre of this phenomenon, a series of wider kinship networks are created, described by those involved as an 'extended family'. These kinship relationships are based on both direct and indirect genetic connections and shared understandings and experiences, out of which new concepts of the family are being defined and negotiated.'

Dr Freeman added: 'Donor siblings have rarely been mentioned in policy discussions about the regulation of gamete donation, beyond concerns about the possibility of unwitting "incestual" relationships between people conceived with the same donor.

'A recent example is the proposal made in a report from the British Fertility Society's (BFS) Working Party on Sperm Donation Services in the UK that the maximum number of families created by a single donor should be raised from the current limit of ten. This was proposed as a means of tackling concerns about falling numbers of donors following the removal of donor anonymity. Despite widespread media attention, the potential psychological effects on donor-conceived offspring of discovering large numbers of genetic siblings in different families was not considered in this debate.

'Part of the reason that there has been limited discussion of donor siblings is that there has been a lack of research in this area. Whilst this current study provides valuable empirical information, it must be highlighted that further research is required into the experiences of those donor offspring who have found, contacted and met large numbers of donor siblings in order to assess the long-term impact on their psychological well-being.'

The study also found differences between types of families had a significant impact on parents' motivations in searching for donor relations. Parents in households without fathers were much more curious about their child's donor and donor siblings.

Dr Freeman said: 'Greater differences were found between one- and two-parent families than between father-present (i.e. heterosexual-couple families) and father-absent families (lone-mother and lesbian-couple families). This is important because, in media and policy discussions, lone mothers and lesbian couples are often grouped together and compared to heterosexual-couple families.'

She continued: 'It is also important to bear in mind that the age and manner in which individuals are told about their donor conception has been found to have a significant impact on how they deal with this information, with those who find

out younger in life experiencing more positive outcomes. This may have a knock-on effect in terms of the experience of contacting donor siblings. In this light, it is important to note that the large majority (97%) of the parents in this study had told, or planned to tell, their offspring about their donor conception, with most having done so at an early age.'

The study is the first large-scale investigation into the experiences of parents of donor-conceived children searching for and contacting their child's donor relations, and it was conducted by one of the world's leading research groups studying embryo, sperm and egg donation and surrogacy. It is one of three papers in the current issue of *Human Reproduction* (a journal of the European Society of Human Reproduction and Embryology) that look at parents' attitudes and experiences towards donors.[2]

One of these papers is an editorial commentary by Dr Pim Janssens, an associate editor of *Human Reproduction*. Writing about Dr Freeman's study, he says: 'Overall, these findings suggest that knowledge of donor sibling families is a good thing, and that disclosure of the donor identity makes sense, and need not be a problem. They also suggest that for many parents and children, having only information about donors is not satisfactory – real encounters are the ultimate desire. Unexpectedly these

findings might also lead us to question the importance of a common family history for the creation of "family feeling". After all, none of the donor families calling their donor sibling relatives shared anything but genes. Nonetheless, many said they felt intuitively bonded.'

References

1 Gamete donation: parents' experiences of searching for their child's donor siblings and donor. *Human Reproduction*, volume 24, issue 3, pages 505-516; doi: 10.1093/humrep/den469.

2 The other two papers are: 'Embryo donation parents' attitudes towards donors: comparison with adoption' (volume 24, issue 3, pages 517-523; doi: 10.1093/humrep/den386) by Fiona MacCallum and 'Colouring the different phases in gamete and embryo donation' (volume 24, issue 3, pages 502-504; doi: 10.1093/humrep/den431) by Pim M.W. Janssens.

24 February 2009

⇨ The above information is reprinted with kind permission from the European Society of Human Reproduction and Embryology. Visit www.eshre.com for more information.

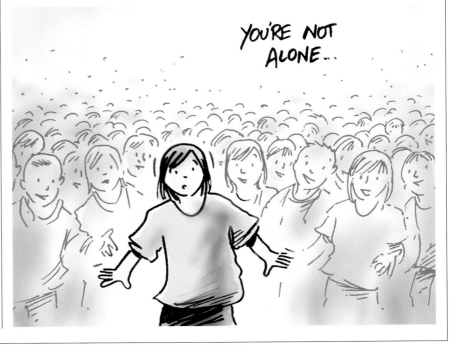

'Saviour siblings'

You may have heard that the law is being changed to allow doctors to help couples create so-called 'saviour siblings': babies that can help cure serious illnesses in their older brothers or sisters. But how does it work, and what can it be used for? We take a look at the science and explain what happens

What are 'saviour siblings'?

For many years, doctors have been able to successfully treat children with certain serious diseases using bone marrow transplants. Bone marrow is a spongy material inside our bones, which makes different types of blood cells. If the bone marrow is damaged by illness, it can no longer make the blood cells the body needs.

A bone marrow transplant involves taking special cells, called stem cells, from the bone marrow of a healthy person and injecting them into the bone marrow of the sick child. Stem cells are able to produce new, healthy blood cells.

It's not new for doctors to use tissue from the brother or sister of a sick child in the hope of curing a serious disease

---

More recently, doctors have started using stem cells from the umbilical cords of newborn babies in a similar way.

But these treatments only work if the bone marrow or stem cells being used are a close match for the cells of the child being treated. The best chance of matching cells comes from a brother or sister (sibling), because they will share the same mixture of genes from the mother and father.

So it's not new for doctors to use tissue from the brother or sister of a sick child in the hope of curing a serious disease. But since 2001, doctors have been able to test the cells of embryos created by IVF, to see whether they are a match for the sick child. This means that, in theory, parents could have babies they have chosen specifically to help their sick child.

These children have been called 'saviour siblings' because they may be able to save the life of their sick older brother or sister.

What conditions can be helped by 'saviour siblings'?

The types of conditions where umbilical cord stem cells or bone marrow is used are mostly blood diseases. These include problems with the immune system, and a type of incurable anaemia where the bone marrow doesn't produce red blood cells. Also, if a child has leukaemia (cancer of the blood) they may need a bone marrow or stem cell transplant to replace the cancerous cells with healthy cells.

What happens to create 'saviour siblings'?

It's quite a complicated process. Here's what needs to happen:
⇨ The sick child's doctors have to agree that stem cells or bone marrow from a brother or sister is the only option for treating the child's illness.
⇨ The child's parents have IVF. They need to produce a lot of embryos to test. So the woman needs to take drugs to make her produce more eggs than normal. The eggs are fertilised by the man's sperm in the laboratory.
⇨ The doctors wait till the embryos are three days old. At this stage they usually consist of eight cells each. They remove one cell from each embryo.
⇨ The cell is tested to see if it's a match for the sick child. If the child has an inherited disease, the cell will also be tested to try to be sure it doesn't have the same disease.

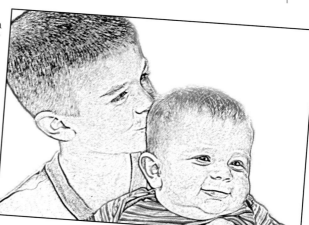

⇨ If an embryo is a good match, it will be implanted into the woman's womb. If this is successful, the embryo will grow into a healthy baby.
⇨ When the baby is born, doctors will collect blood from the umbilical cord. This blood may be given to the sick child as a blood transfusion. Or, if the sick child needs a bone marrow transplant, the doctors will wait until the baby is old enough to take some of its healthy bone marrow and give it to the sick child.

How well does it work?

We don't know. This is a new technique and it has only been tried a few times. Many things can go wrong:
⇨ The embryos produced by IVF may not be a good match. IVF is a difficult and expensive process. Parents may not be able to go through it enough times to product a matching embryo.
⇨ IVF may not work. The embryo put into the woman's womb might not grow into a healthy baby.
⇨ The test may not be completely accurate, so the baby might not be a good match after all.

Because it is such a new technique, we don't know whether there might be long-term effects for the baby. So far, it seems that embryos that carry on developing after having a cell removed grow into normal children.

Why are MPs changing the law?

There are strict laws governing what fertility clinics can and can't do. But science has moved on since these laws were passed in 1990. The current law doesn't say whether fertility clinics can test embryos to create 'saviour siblings'. Individual cases have been tested in the courts, and some clinics have been allowed to do testing, but only in these specific cases.

The bill being debated at the moment says that licensed clinics should be allowed to test embryos for tissue matching, to help produce a 'saviour sibling', so long as certain safeguards are met.

MPs have voted in favour of this part of the bill, which is likely to become law in April 2009.

From:

⇨ Department of Health, *Human Fertilisation and Embryology Bill 2008*, available at http://www.commonsleader.gov.uk/output/page2162.asp
⇨ Human Fertilisation and Embry-

ology Authority: *Report on pre-implantation tissue typing*, July 2004, available at http://www.hfea.gov.uk/en/494.html
⇨ Human Genetics Commission, *Pre-implantation Genetic Diagnosis*, available at http://www.hgc.gov.uk/UploadDocs/Contents/Documents/PGD%20Template.doc
22 May 2008

⇨ The above information is reprinted with kind permission from the BMJ Publishing Group. Visit www.bmj.com for more information.
© BMJ Publishing Group

My Jamie is not a 'designer baby'. . .

. . .he has given his brother a new life

The film of Jodi Picoult's My Sister's Keeper *is set to reignite the ethical debate over embryo selection. Here one family tell why they chose to have a child whose stem cells have saved his brother from a nightmare existence of transfusions and injections.*

Michelle Whitaker visibly winces at the term designer baby. 'Horrible,' she says. 'Like "harvest baby" or "spare parts baby". It's just wrong.

'What did we design about Jamie? Not his eye colour, his hair colour, his IQ, his height.'

So what about the term 'saviour sibling'?

'Well, he is a saviour sibling, and he's very proud of that,' she says, watching her youngest child playing in their Derbyshire back garden. Jamie celebrated his sixth birthday last week, a joyous occasion marked by a party at Laser Quest with his brother, Charlie, ten, sister Emily, seven, and friends.

Such normality contrasts greatly with the day he was born, delivered in the midst of raging controversy over embryo testing. Chosen through pre-implantation genetic diagnosis (PIGD) as a perfect tissue match for

Charlie, who had been diagnosed with rare Diamond Blackfan anaemia, the method of Jamie's conception and birth was condemned by some campaigners as another step along a 'stem cell-paved road to hell'.

The release this week of the film *My Sister's Keeper* is set to inflame that debate again and throw the spotlight back on families such as the Whitakers. Set in America and starring Cameron Diaz, the film is based on a novel by Jodi Picoult. The central character, Anna, is genetically selected to save her leukaemia-stricken sister, Kate. Like Jamie, she has been specially picked for this task. Kate is infused with precious umbilical cord blood, rich in hematopoietic stem cells (HSCs) from her baby sibling, in the hope that it will cure her.

But here is where the Whitakers' reality and the film's fiction part company. For, as Anna grows older, more is demanded of her by

parents desperate to save Kate's life. Eventually, Anna sues for medical emancipation from her parents, and the right to decide how her body should be used.

> **The method of Jamie's conception and birth was condemned by some campaigners as another step along a 'stem cell-paved road to hell'**

Fiction it may be, but Michelle, a former medical secretary, fears the film will serve to harden attitudes towards the methods used to save Charlie. 'It has taken a situation like ours, and pushed and pushed it to the absolute extremes. People are going to think, "Ah, that's why people are doing it."

'It's going to bring the "spare parts" baby debate back again. It's so dramatic,' adds Michelle, 37, who has read the novel. 'The things that are described, well, they just wouldn't be allowed to happen in this country.'

It's a hellish plot, an ethical and

moral rollercoaster. That's not to say the Whitakers cannot identify with parts of it. 'It was a fight all the way. It was hell on earth for this family,' says Michelle's husband, Jayson, 39, the managing director of an energy company. In the end, it was a hell that drove them from Britain to America in search of help.

It is hard to believe that now, as their three children scramble excitedly around the garden of their family home, a renovated cottage near Chesterfield with breathtaking views across the countryside, with their pet labrador and terrier in tow. Dinner is on. Notes pinned to the kitchen noticeboard testify to a busy life of Scouts, dentist's appointments, homework to be done, party invitations – the normal, semi-chaotic life enjoyed by millions of families throughout Britain.

But it didn't used to be like that. Looking at photographs, Michelle and Jayson can now see that Charlie was not a normal newborn. 'He looks grey,' says Michelle, though as a first-time mother she thought, perhaps, this was what he was supposed to look like.

It was not until he was 12 weeks that Diamond Blackfan anaemia, a life-threatening disease that stops the body producing red blood cells, was diagnosed. They were told: 'Your child has DBA. This is the prognosis. This is the treatment. Go away and think about it.'

But the prognosis was uncertain. Few in Britain had experience of it. Jayson found himself on the phone for hours to parents of sufferers in America. As for treatment, it would mean a lifetime of blood transfusions – one every three weeks – plus daily injections of Desferal, a drug to prevent the iron overload from transfusions damaging his vital organs. 'This can't be it,' Jayson protested at the time. 'It can't just be transfusions for the rest of his life. There must be something we can do.'

'I cried my eyes out. I really did. I thought, "Why us? Why not somebody else?" I was heartbroken,' says Michelle.

So began a reality far removed from their dreams of parenthood. Charlie spent more time in hospital than out. Apart from the transfusions, he was regularly admitted with infections. Then there were the daily injections. 'We had to stick a needle in his stomach every night, and hook him up to a pump for 12 hours,' says Michelle. 'I couldn't do it. Jayson did it, because he was stronger. And as Charlie got older and started talking, he would be crying: "Please don't hurt me. You don't love me. Why are you hurting me?" I just couldn't cope with that.'

One consultant seemed to offer hope. There could be a cure, they were told, but it would involve a transplant. The trouble was, Charlie had no siblings. The Whitakers had

always wanted a large family. 'Five,' they chime. Today, they have four – three of their own and a little girl they are fostering. But back then, there were concerns. They wondered if they could be carriers of a gene that causes DBA. They weren't. The cause of Charlie's illness was not genetic but a 'sporadic mutation'. Their chances of having another DBA baby were one in 50. They decided to risk it and conceived Emily naturally.

It was just before Emily was born that they heard of the case of Molly Nash, a girl from Minnesota born with Fanconi anaemia, an often fatal genetic disease, whose parents' decision to chose a 'tissue-match' embryo as their second child – a sibling to help cure her – caused a global media sensation.

Just in case, the Whitakers decided to have Emily's cord blood stored. In the end, she turned out not to be a perfect match, but any disappointment was overwhelmed by the sheer relief that she was not suffering from DBA.

At around the same time, the Human Fertilisation and Embryology Authority (HFEA) was testing the water on embryo selection. In the first decision of its kind, it had given the go-ahead to Raj and Shahana Hashmi, from Leeds, to use PIGD to have a baby that would help cure their son, Zain, who was born with the blood disorder beta thalassaemia.

The decision provoked outrage from some quarters. Josephine Quintavalle, from Comment on Reproductive Ethics, successfully sued the HFEA for acting unlawfully, though that ruling was overturned in the court of appeal and by the law lords.

So it was against this backdrop that the Whitakers approached Dr Mohamed Taranissi, a leading fertility specialist, for help. But, while he agreed, the HFEA said no. Jayson believes the HFEA's decision was swayed by the legal battle over the Hashmi family. 'They wouldn't listen to us. They wouldn't listen to our specialists, even though we begged them.' They refused the application on the grounds that, as Charlie's DBA was not genetic, the embryo itself would not benefit from screening. The Whitakers responded by

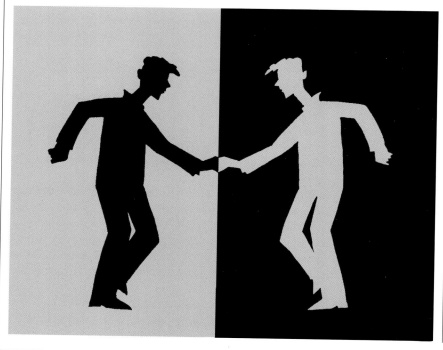

boarding a plane for Chicago. 'There was lots of debate when Jamie was born, that he's going to be totally screwed up in the head because he's a "saviour sibling", a "spare parts" baby. It's all rubbish,' says Michelle. 'It's how you go about bringing a child up. We say to him he should have "Made in America" tattooed on his bottom. He knows how he was made, and why he was made.'

With the HFEA's refusal, the genetic screening and implantation of a tissue-match embryo was performed in America where the rules were more relaxed. But, with just a three-week window (they had to be back in Britain for Charlie's transfusions), and flying to the US with two small children and a box full of needles and medicine immediately after the 11 September attacks, it was an ordeal. Then, when

Jamie was born the family had to wait 12 months in case he, too, showed symptoms of DBA.

Five years after his transplant, Charlie is still clear of DBA. And the bond between the two brothers is clear. 'If anything, it's Emily, not Jamie, who feels left out, because she couldn't help,' says Michelle.

Tucking into her roast chicken dinner, Emily proffers shyly: 'Jamie says that Charlie needed boys' blood, that's why.'

'No,' counters Jamie. 'He needed a match. It was easy-peasy,' he adds.

In *My Sister's Keeper*, much is made of the isolation that Kate's two siblings feel. There is no evidence of that in the Whitaker household. Jayson wouldn't read the book and he has no intention of seeing the film. Michelle has not yet decided.

'We didn't have any hate mail, but people thought we were actually taking Jamie's bone marrow and bits of Jamie. It was just the cord blood that was required. Nothing else. It's a waste product thrown out at birth.

'It never crossed my mind that we would have to use Jamie again, and it was never mentioned to us, either.'

Even if Charlie were to have a relapse? 'Well, I don't know,' she admits. 'But that wouldn't be our decision. It would be up to the courts. Not like in this film, where they just used that child for everything without even consulting her. In real life, it's not like that. That's what people probably won't understand.'

21 June 2009

Row over clinic that offers eye, skin and hair colour

A Los Angeles clinic is offering the ultimate in designer babies. Want a son with brown eyes, black hair and a dark complexion? Or a pale-skinned, blonde, green-eyed daughter?

The Fertility Institutes clinic has just started offering prospective parents the opportunity to select physical traits of future offspring thanks to 'cosmetic medicine'.

But other fertility experts are outraged that the clinic is seeking to capitalise on dramatic advances in embryo cell analysis designed to identify dangerous diseases and defects in the unborn.

By Philip Sherwell in New York

They are angered that the bespoke baby in vitro fertilisation service is distracting public attention from how the pioneering medical technology can have children free of debilitating genetic conditions.

Clinic director Dr Jeff Steinberg, who as a young medic was part of the team involved in the birth in Britain in 1978 of Louise Brown, the world's first test tube baby, is undeterred.

'It's incredibly exciting,' he told the *Sunday Telegraph*. 'I live in LA and everyone here wants to have a straight nose and high cheekbones and are perfectly happy to pay for cosmetic surgery.

'I understand the trepidation and concerns, but we cannot escape the fact that science is moving forward. If I have to get smacked around by people

who think it is inappropriate, then I'm willing to live with that.'

> **The Fertility Institutes clinic has just started offering prospective parents the opportunity to select physical traits of future offspring thanks to 'cosmetic medicine'**

Dr Steinberg's clinic, already the world's largest provider of the controversial process of gender choice, has received 'five or six' requests from couples for the new service which involves embryo selection, not genetic modification.

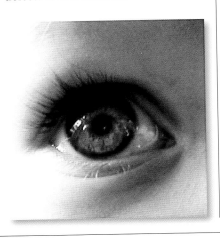

He expects the first trait selection baby to be born next year and the cost for the process to be about $18,000 (£12,700) – the same bottom line for parents who choose their baby's sex.

The ground-breaking science is based on a procedure known as pre-implantation genetic diagnosis (PGD) that for years has allowed doctors to identify potentially lethal diseases and conditions in embryos.

But scientists have recently made startling advances in their ability to analyse the make-up of a single cell – the size of one-thousandth of a grain of sand – taken from a three-day-old embryo.

At a meeting of the American Society of Human Genetics late last year, William Kearns, a leading medical geneticist, outlined how he had managed to obtain sufficient DNA from the cell to identify thousands of characteristics from the embryo.

Dr Kearns explained the technique for medical purposes, but Dr Steinberg quickly spotted other uses. 'It's a bit like Google Earth technology,' he said. 'You used to be able to see a street from space and now we can see through the front window.'

He said parents might seek the clinic's services for both medical and cosmetic reasons. Some couples might, for example, already have a child with a skin cancer such as melanoma and want their next baby to have a darker complexion for medical reasons. But others might just want a blonde girl with green eyes. 'Is it medical or cosmetic or both?' he asked.

His proposal to offer trait selection has outraged Dr Kearns. 'I won't sell my soul for any amount,' he said. 'Steinberg has jumped on my research but I'm totally against this. My goal is to screen embryos to help couples have healthy babies free of genetic diseases. Traits are not diseases.'

And Mark Hughes, one of the 'fathers' of PGD, is just as bitterly opposed to the trait selection service on offer from the Fertility Institutes. 'It's ridiculous and irresponsible,' said the director of Genesis Genetics in Detroit. 'There are thousands of desperate couples who have no hope of having healthy children without this technology, and here we are talking about this.'

The row about the selection of these physical traits is doubtless only a taste of the furore that will follow if scientists are able to work out which human genome combinations predicate height, sporting prowess and perhaps the ultimate taboo, intelligence.

Britain, in common with most European nations, has banned the process of gender selection, although some British couples determined to choose a boy or girl have travelled to countries where the process is not illegal.

The American Society for Reproductive Medicine has issued guidelines against gender selection – trait selection is so new that it has not yet been considered – but it has fiercely opposed the sort of government regulations that are imposed in Europe.

In the wake of the 'octomom' saga, in which 33-year-old mother-of-six Nadja Suleman recently gave birth to another eight babies after IVF at a different Los Angeles clinic, the Fertility Institutes offer has heightened the controversy about whether the industry should be regulated.

'In the US, we're in the Wild West on this,' said Marcy Darnovsky, director of the California-based Centre for Genetics and Society.

'The concern is that we'll be creating a society with new sorts of discrimination. Now it's eyes and hair colour. What happens if it's height and intelligence? Some parents may have qualms about that, but still feel under pressure to go down that route.'

But Dr Steinberg said that he recalled walking into the car park after the birth of Louise Brown three decades ago and finding a scrawled note on his windshield bearing the message 'test tube babies have no soul'.

He added: 'It was new, people didn't understand it and they were afraid. Now IVF is not even a cocktail party curiosity.'

28 February 2009

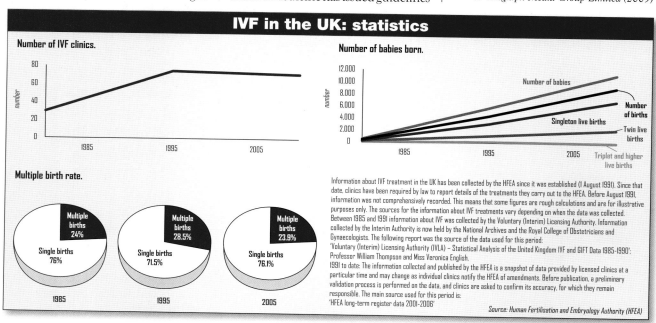

IVF in the UK: statistics

Number of IVF clinics.

Number of babies born.

Number of babies

Number of births

Singleton live births

Twin live births

Triplet and higher live births

Multiple birth rate.

Multiple births 24% / Single births 76% — 1985

Multiple births 28.5% / Single births 71.5% — 1995

Multiple births 23.9% / Single births 76.1% — 2005

Information about IVF treatment in the UK has been collected by the HFEA since it was established (1 August 1991). Since that date, clinics have been required by law to report details of the treatments they carry out to the HFEA. Before August 1991, information was not comprehensively recorded. This means that some figures are rough calculations and are for illustrative purposes only. The sources for the information about IVF treatments vary depending on when the data was collected. Between 1985 and 1991 information about IVF was collected by the Voluntary (Interim) Licensing Authority. Information collected by the Interim Authority is now held by the National Archives and the Royal College of Obstetricians and Gynaecologists. The following report was the source of the data used for this period:
'Voluntary (Interim) Licensing Authority (IVLA) – Statistical Analysis of the United Kingdom IVF and GIFT Data 1985-1990'; Professor William Thompson and Miss Veronica English.
1991 to date: The information collected and published by the HFEA is a snapshot of data provided by licensed clinics at a particular time and may change as individual clinics notify the HFEA of amendments. Before publication, a preliminary validation process is performed on the data, and clinics are asked to confirm its accuracy, for which they remain responsible. The main source used for this period is:
'HFEA long-term register data 2001-2006'

Source: Human Fertilisation and Embryology Authority (HFEA)

Stem cell research: hope or hype?

Exploration of the ethical questions

Introduction

Adult stem cells can be obtained relatively safely from adults who have given consent for such procedures or from children whose parents/guardians have consented on their behalf. Consequently, the ethical challenges posed by stem cell research relate almost exclusively to embryonic stem cells. The harvesting of embryonic stem cells currently requires the destruction of embryos and this is unacceptable to those who believe life begins at conception. Therefore, this information will largely focus on the ethics of embryonic stem cell research.

Should stem cells from umbilical cord blood be stored?

As mentioned above, adult stem cell research is relatively uncontroversial. However, one area which has raised ethical questions is the storage of babies' umbilical cord blood.

Since 1988 it has been shown that adult stem cells present in the blood of the umbilical cord can be used for transplantation in a number of genetic and blood diseases as well as immune deficiencies, e.g. leukaemia. After transplantation the stem cells repopulate the bone marrow of the patient, providing a source of blood cells. Blood from the umbilical cord and placenta can be collected during or immediately after the birth of a child. After collection the cord is reduced in volume, frozen at a controlled rate and stored in liquid nitrogen at −196°C. Commercial companies now offer parents the opportunity to store their own baby's cord blood, in case the child or his/her siblings ever develop a disease that could in the future be treated by cord blood stem cell transplantation. There is currently a debate about whether storing a child's umbilical cord blood is a worthwhile investment for future healthcare or an expensive procedure, which might never prove beneficial.

Concerns have been raised regarding the promises made about the potential for cord blood transplants to treat a number of diseases for which there is, at present, no medical evidence. Therefore, opponents argue that the State should not be paying for storage when there are no proven benefits. Opponents also argue that the chances of umbilical cord blood stem cells ever being needed by all of the families who store it are very small.

Therefore, they raise concerns regarding the commercial storage of umbilical cord blood. They state that allowing parents who can afford to pay for storage to do so would force those who cannot afford to store their babies' cord blood to feel unduly guilty.

Proponents argue that given the nature of recent scientific advances there is a reasonable likelihood that umbilical cord blood stem cells will become of significant medical value in the coming years. Some argue that the State should put resources into establishing a national umbilical cord blood bank, similar to the national blood bank, where everyone can donate their babies' cord blood and where cells are shared with patients based on medical need. Others argue that parents who wish to pay commercial companies to store umbilical cord blood should not be prevented from doing so. They state that umbilical cord blood storage is akin to other forms of medical insurance, which might never be needed, and that parents who can afford to do so should be free to make an autonomous decision, i.e. a decision free from external influences.

What is the moral status of the embryo?

Moral status refers to the moral value we give to the various beings with which we share the world, i.e. fellow humans and other animal species. Moral status also refers to the rights, if any, to which various beings are entitled.

There is a wide spectrum of opinions in relation to the moral status of embryos. There are those who believe that an embryo has full moral status and is deserving of the same rights, protection and respect as an adult human being from the moment of conception. Stem cell research involving the destruction of human embryos, therefore, is

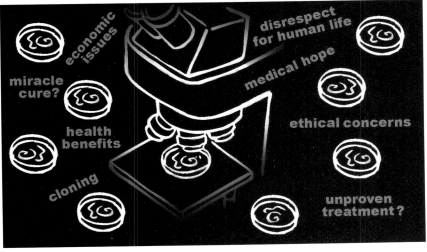

morally unacceptable for those who hold this view.

There are also those who believe that embryos gradually gain moral status as they develop (known as the gradualist approach). For instance, the implantation of an embryo into the mother's womb is regarded as a critical step. Others consider the appearance of a nervous system or the ability of the foetus to feel pain as critical points in development. Therefore, those who hold the gradualist view consider that the therapeutic possibilities offered by embryonic stem cell research may outweigh the infringements of the respect and dignity of the embryo.

The harvesting of embryonic stem cells currently requires the destruction of embryos and this is unacceptable to those who believe life begins at conception

Alternatively, there are those who consider embryos to be balls of cells, which do not have rights and require no legal protection. This group, therefore, have no moral objection to embryonic stem cell research being undertaken.

Is an embryo a person?
Related to the debate regarding the moral status of embryos is the debate about personhood. There are numerous opinions regarding its definition and onset. On one side there are those who argue that two conditions are required for personhood to be in place, namely the ability to reason and the capacity for self-awareness, which both require a certain level of brain function. They say that because embryos do not have such capacities, they should not be afforded personhood or full moral status. However, on the other side it has been argued that some people, e.g. the severely mentally incapacitated and very young babies, would not have the capabilities required for

personhood, yet society still considers them worthy of full moral status.

Does the potential of embryos affect their moral status?
The potentiality of embryos is also an important consideration when discussing moral status. Some commentators have expressed the view that embryos are due considerable moral status. They state that while embryos are not yet considered persons, they are part of the human family and that, if not interfered with, they have the potential to develop into persons.

Others who argue that a being's potential does not always translate into reality, dispute the potentiality argument. For example, many of us have the potential to become criminals, yet it would not be considered reasonable to treat us as such unless we actually fulfil that potential. This group argue that moral status and its associated rights and protections should be based on the actual rather than the potential properties of a being. Others have argued that since the rate of natural embryo loss, before and after implantation in the womb is somewhere between 30-80%, the potential that embryos have to develop is not very strong. Consequently, it has been argued that this weakens the potentiality argument.

Should embryos produced but not used during IVF be used for stem cell research?
Embryos, which are produced during in-vitro fertilisation (IVF), may not always be implanted, e.g. a couple may have completed their family or may have separated. These unused embryos might be placed in storage, allowed to perish, donated to other couples or donated for research. Proponents of embryonic stem cell research argue that embryos produced but not used during IVF should be made available for use in research. They claim that there is a moral onus on society to use these embryos, which would otherwise be allowed to perish, for research into debilitating or life-threatening illnesses and injuries. However, those who afford full moral status to embryos reject this argument

and compare research on embryos produced but not used during IVF to performing research on terminally ill people without their consent. They also argue that allowing embryos to perish is not equivalent to actively destroying them.

Should embryos be created specifically for stem cell research?
Therapeutic cloning is the process by which human embryos are created in order to obtain embryonic stem cells for research purposes. Proponents of embryonic stem cell research argue that the creation of embryos specifically for research should be permitted. Some argue that because sperm and egg are not combined to create these embryos, such embryos do not have the same moral status as embryos produced but not used during IVF. However, opponents say that the creation of embryos specifically for research represents disrespect for human life because creating embryos, which are never intended for implantation, treats the embryo merely as a means to an end. They also dismiss the creation of embryos specifically for research as premature when there are other more ethical sources of stem cells available, e.g. adult stem cells. Others fear that allowing the use of therapeutic cloning to create embryos for research would set science on a 'slippery slope' towards reproductive cloning.

Where will the eggs, necessary for conducting therapeutic cloning, come from?
In order to undertake therapeutic cloning scientists would need to have access to a supply of eggs. Concerns have been raised regarding the procurement of these eggs. The harvesting of eggs from women is a procedure not without risk, which could result in ovarian hyperstimulation syndrome, i.e. ovaries become enlarged and fluid accumulates in the abdomen causing pain, nausea, breathing difficulties which can lead to hospitalisation and, in extreme cases, death. There are also fears that significant financial incentives may be offered to women in order to encourage them to donate their eggs

for research. Opponents argue that paying women for egg donation would lead to the commercialisation of the human body by placing a monetary value on body parts. Furthermore, there are fears that paying women for their eggs could lead to the exploitation of the economically disadvantaged as only those in need would be persuaded to take risks for financial gain. However, others argue that in the interest of personal autonomy women should be free to choose whether or not they wish to undergo medical procedures in return for payment.

An alternative source of stem cells to adult tissue and embryos is the creation of human-animal hybrids or chimeras. The word chimera refers to a Greek mythological creature, which had the head of a lion, the body of a goat and the tail of a snake. Human-animal chimeras are created through the fusion of human cells and animal eggs. Proponents argue that using human-animal embryos, would negate the need to use eggs from women to produce embryos for stem cell research. Opponents raise concerns that the creation of chimeras for the purpose of stem cell research will blur the distinction between humans and animals. They say that there is a significant 'yuk' factor associated with mixing elements of humans and animals and that the public might view the research as 'Frankenstein science'. There are also concerns that the mixing of different species will increase the risk of transferring animal diseases to humans.

Should the Irish Health Service provide possible future treatments developed from embryonic stem cell research to Irish citizens?

There is currently a debate regarding the decisions faced by future policy makers in the event of therapies being developed from embryonic stem cell research. Some people argue that it would be morally inconsistent for future governments to provide treatments derived from embryonic stem cell research when the research itself is not permitted here. They argue that making treatments available here

would be akin to being complicit in the destruction of the embryos used for the research. On the other hand, some argue that if treatments become available the damage will have already been done and that the therapies could be used to treat sick members of society. They argue that it would be unethical of society not to provide the treatments. Proponents also argue that the provision of treatments derived from embryonic stem cell research would depend on how far removed the treatments would be from the initial research, e.g. whether the treatment consisted of embryonic stem cells or was a synthetic product based on research involving embryonic stem cells.

⇨ The above information is reprinted with kind permission from the Irish Council for Bioethics. Visit www.bioethics.i.e. for more information.

© Irish Council for Bioethics

Pope slams embryo research as immoral

Information from the Christian Institute

Pope Benedict has hit out against destructive experiments on human embryos and called for more work to be done in the ethical field of adult stem cells.

The comments come in a strongly worded Vatican document on reproductive science – the first for 20 years – personally approved by the Pope.

The report says the morning-after pill and other measures which can act to destroy an embryo by preventing it from implanting in a womb are 'gravely immoral'.

It also condemns the creation of 'designer babies' and embryos that are part animal, part human. The creation of animal-human embryos for research was recently made lawful in Britain.

The Vatican document confirms the Roman Catholic Church's position that all human life deserves respect 'from the very first stages of its existence and can never be reduced merely to a group of cells'.

The report says that stem cell research should be encouraged if tissues are obtained from adults, umbilical cord blood or foetuses that have died naturally.

There have been many reports recently highlighting medical breakthroughs using adult stem cells.

Most recently, in November, British scientists successfully used adult stem cells to create a replacement windpipe for a mother-of-two.

The breakthrough came just weeks after Parliament passed new legislation liberalising embryo research, despite hearing evidence that time and funding would be better spent on work using adult stem cells.

16 December 2008

⇨ The above information is reprinted with kind permission from the Christian Institute. Visit www.christian.org.uk for more information.

© Christian Institute

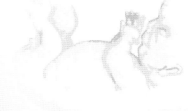

A humanist discussion of embryo research

Information from the British Humanist Association

Humanist ethics

Humanists seek to live good lives without religious or superstitious beliefs. They use reason, experience and respect for others when thinking about moral issues, not obedience to dogmatic rules. Humanists promote happiness and fulfilment in this life because they believe it's the only one we have. When deciding whether something is right or wrong, humanists consider the evidence and the probable effects of choices.

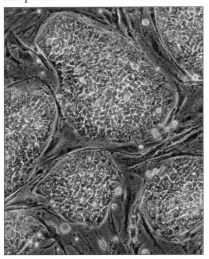

Human embryonic stem cells

Embryo research is a subject that demonstrates the difficulties of rigid unchanging rules in moral decision making. Medical science has advanced to the point where we have options that were unthinkable even a few years ago and where old rules cannot cope with new facts.

21st-century medicine could be transformed by research into using human embryos as a source of tissue-repairing cells, often called 'therapeutic cloning'. This is different from 'reproductive cloning', where cloned embryos would be grown from a cell taken from one individual and then implanted in a womb where they would develop into near replicas of their one parent.

Therapeutic cloning

Using 'stem cells' from very early embryos (under 14 days of age), which are capable of developing into any of the specialised cells of the body, replacement tissue could be grown in the laboratory and used to cure many currently incurable conditions, avoiding the problem of immune rejection. But the use of human embryos raises ethical questions and provokes much opposition, particularly from religious and anti-abortion groups, who use similar arguments to those used to oppose contraception and abortion to object to the exploitation of a living human embryo. Opponents also fear that embryo research for therapeutic purposes is a 'slippery slope' that will lead to the cloning of human beings. Some religious groups accuse medical researchers of 'playing God'.

Humanists respect life, but are not religious and so do not worry about 'playing God' or believe in 'the sanctity of life'. (Human beings have been 'playing God' for a long time, intervening beneficially in reproductive and medical processes.) For humanists the most important consideration in ethical questions on life and death is the quality of life of the individual person. In the case of embryo research, humanists would focus on two issues: whether an embryo is indeed a person, and whether the research on and subsequent use of embryo cells would do more good than harm.

Is an embryo a person?

At the early stage where research is focused, an embryo has few of the characteristics we associate with a person. It is a fertilised human egg, with the capacity to develop into a person, but its cells have not yet begun to form into specialist cells that would form particular parts of the body (which is why they are potentially so useful). There is no brain, no self-

---

Questions to think about

⇨ Do you think an early stage embryo is a human being with human rights?

⇨ How big is a 14-day-old embryo? What does it look like? (Ask your Biology teacher.)

⇨ Find out what use(s) might be made of cloned embryo cells.

⇨ Find out what the law on embryo research is now, and if there are any plans to change it. Do you support change? Give reasons for your viewpoint.

⇨ Find out who supports embryo research and who opposes it, and why.

⇨ Do we need more people?

⇨ Do we need more of specific kinds of people?

⇨ Do we need them so much that we are prepared to take risks in order to produce them?

⇨ How are you deciding your answers to these questions? What principles and arguments influence your answers?

⇨ How is the humanist view on this issue similar to that of other worldviews you have come across? How is it different?

awareness (or consciousness), no way of feeling pain or emotion, so an early stage embryo cannot suffer.

Should we consider embryo donors?

Fertility treatments produce many of the 'spare embryos' that would be used, and parents might feel some attachment to these or concern or guilt about what happens to them. It would seem right to inform them fully about what might happen to their embryos, and to take their feelings into account. If they do not consent to donating their embryos for medical research, they should not be used. On the other hand, spare embryos are routinely disposed of at the moment, so already they are not treated as human beings, and parents do not seem unduly concerned. Donors may even prefer their embryos to be used to help someone, rather than wasted, just as many people consent to organ donation.

So, should we allow therapeutic cloning?

If an embryo's cells can be used to alleviate human suffering, the good consequences seem to outweigh the harmful ones, as long as the legal cut off point for research is sufficiently early. Do embryos being produced specially for research and therapeutic purposes by IVF in the laboratory raise any new moral issues? The consequences seem to be much the same, so a humanist would probably think not. So most humanists would support therapeutic cloning, because they do not consider very early embryos to be people, unlike some religious people.

Is this a slippery slope? Will we be cloning human beings next?

It is often argued that therapeutic cloning will inevitably lead to reproductive cloning – a classic 'slippery slope' argument. Many scientists (over half a small sample polled by the *Independent* in August 2000) think that therapeutic cloning will develop research techniques and skills that will inevitably be used for human reproductive cloning. There does indeed appear to be a technical slippery slope between therapeutic

cloning and reproductive cloning, which has already proved possible in animals (in the case of Dolly the sheep). However, there are also very clear differences between the two, which make it possible to distinguish between them morally – it is not a moral slippery slope. New cures for disease are needed and the consequences of producing new treatments seem, on balance, to be good. But in an over-populated world new ways of creating human beings are not needed, and the consequences of producing human beings by cloning might not be good at all.

Cloned human beings might suffer from unintended physical side-effects of the process, such as premature ageing or infertility, or other abnormalities, and we might decide that it would be unethical to grow human beings experimentally to the point where this could be detected. It is possible that cloned children could suffer psychologically – as do some adopted children or those born as a result of IVF. In many ways cloning seems like a vanity project: a parent would have to be very confident of his own qualities to want to produce a near identical child, and the expectations the parent would have of the child might hinder its healthy emotional development. For these reasons, humanists would probably oppose reproductive cloning.

Some of the fears raised by cloning do seem exaggerated – it would be a costly, slow and unlikely way to raise a super-fit army of Olympic athletes or scientific geniuses – selection from the existing population, training, and education would be much more cost effective. Fears that children would be absolutely identical to their parent, a younger twin, in effect, seem unfounded when we take into account the vital role of environment and upbringing in making us who we are: the child's experience of life would be very different from its parent's.

But even if some fears are irrational, we would need very good reasons to embark on an experiment that we might not fully know the results of for several decades. Knowing how to do something does not mean that we necessarily have to do it. Human beings have all kinds of knowledge and capabilities that we have decided it would be better not to use, for example, the USA and the former USSR have stockpiles of nuclear weapons that could wipe out life on Earth, but have chosen not to deploy them. Reproductive cloning might be another example. It is worth remembering that it not for scientists alone to decide how to use their research – it is a decision for society, and that means all of us.

With thanks to Professor Lewis Wolpert, CBE, FRS

⇨ The above information is reprinted with kind permission from the British Humanist Association. Visit www.humanism.org.uk for more information.

© *British Humanist Association*

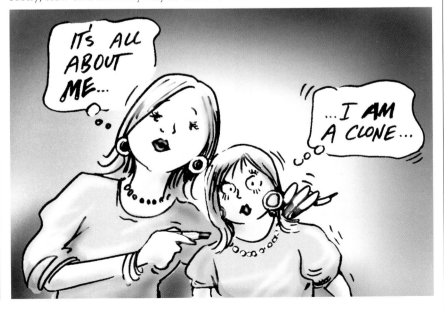

Victory for ethics?

Embryonic-like stem cells breakthrough

The UK media is reporting a stem cell breakthrough that could end the ethical battle over the use of human embryos.

Some facts

The most recent breakthrough in the stem cell technology relates to induced pluripotent stem cells (iPS cells),* cells which are embryonic-type but do not require the destruction of human embryos.

This new process of deriving such stem cells was announced first in 2007, in Japan and the US, and was immediately taken up across the world as an exciting development *per se* and which could as well eliminate ethical concerns regarding the use of embryos.

In layman's terms this is an adult cell manipulated to go back in time to the state of an embryonic stem cell, but not to the state of an embryo. It has then to be re-directed to create the specific tissue required for regenerative therapy.

This new technology was immediately seen as having scientific advantages over the use of human embryos, as the desired cells could be created from the patients themselves, thus providing perfectly matching tissue. When human embryos are involved, on the other hand, the resulting cells could never be a perfect match, and risks of immune rejection would have to be addressed.

This week's exciting news of further progress with iPS cells is in relationship to a safety issue associated with the initial technology. A gene-carrying virus was used to derive the first iPS cells and it was proving difficult to remove this virus, which would have prohibited any chance of moving this research towards therapy.

But teams from the UK and Canada have now revealed that they have solved the problem by using a new process, which introduces the necessary genes without the virus. The genes are then removed and the resulting cells are healthy and intact and behave the same way as embryonic stem cells derived from human embryos.

The way forward

The task now for scientists is to find the way to turn these embryonic-type stem cells into the various cell types required for therapy, and to ensure that if implanted they do not grow out of control and cause tumours. This is not a problem exclusive to this new type of embryonic stem cell, however. It exists equally for those derived from human embryos as well. Much research still needs to be done to harness the full potential of these cells, to ensure that they differentiate successfully and safely.

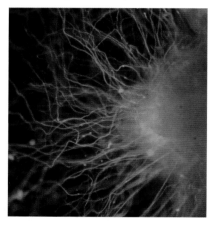

Human embryonic stem cell - a nerve cell

Cures?

We have a duty to the patients waiting for cures not to over-hype new developments in the field of stem cell regeneration, whatever type is under scrutiny. We must accept, however, that whilst adult stem cell therapies have been applied successfully – in some cases for decades – to thousands of patients, the field of embryonic stem cell therapy is still in its early stages.

Caution aside, the new development still makes a colossal leap forward in stem cell regenerative medicine. That no human embryos are sacrificed in the process is a great joy to CORE and to many others, including a considerable number of scientists who do research on the human embryo but have confessed they would prefer not to.

It is appropriate to remind the Human Fertilisation & Embryology Authority that research on the human embryo in the United Kingdom can only take place if it can be shown to be necessary. It is high time for some serious rethinking on their part when they issue or renew licences involving the human embryo.

Embryonic-type cells have been derived successfully and safely from adult tissue

Not only does this current breakthrough solve the big ethical issue of use of the human embryo but it is also the better way forward from a purely scientific viewpoint. This new technology would provide the best tissue match for transplant, derived as it is directly from the patient.

By all accounts, it is also a relatively simple technique, efficient, and within the capabilities of most laboratory facilities.

Verdict?

This is ethical stem cell research we can all agree on. Embryonic-type cells have been derived successfully and safely from adult tissue without involving human embryos.

This is very good news and takes much of the battle out of the stem cell debate.

* *http://news.bbc.co.uk/2/hi/health/7914976.stm*
2 March 2009

⇨ The above information is reprinted with kind permission from Comment on Reproductive Ethics (CORE). Visit www.corethics.org for more.
© *Comment on Reproductive Ethics (CORE)*

Can sperm really be created in a laboratory?

By Sarah Boseley

Anybody who has, for whatever reason, dreamed of a world without men in the past probably looked to the cloners to make it happen. Few would have imagined it might one day be possible to create human sperm in a laboratory, but that is now the proud claim of Professor Karim Nayernia of the North East England Stem Cell Institute.

It is a claim that immediately hit controversy. Allan Pacey of the University of Sheffield, a sperm biologist of 20 years' standing, declared he was unconvinced. Azim Surani, a professor of physiology and reproduction at Cambridge University, said they were 'sperm-like cells' and 'a long way from being authentic sperm cells'.

Discovering how to make sperm will teach us more about sperm malfunction, and therefore could help treat infertile men

Reactions two years ago, when the same team not only grew mouse sperm from embryonic cells but used it to produce baby mice, were somewhat warmer, which perhaps says something about the sensitivities around the creation of human sperm. Pacey said at the time that the mouse experiment would be 'very useful to study the basic biology of sperm production'.

Using technology to produce the essence of human life is a sensitive matter: the baby mice all died after a few months. And while the Newcastle scientists have categorically ruled out the use of their manufactured sperm for reproduction and say they understand people's concerns, the very notion that human sperm have been created from stem cells has taken anxieties to a new level.

'The law specifically does not allow artificially created sperm to be used to fertilise an egg for the sake of reproduction,' says Professor Peter Braude, head of the department of women's health in the division of reproduction and endocrinology at King's College London. And even if the law is changed, he asks, 'What experiments are you going to do to make it safe?' Citing Dolly the Sheep, Braude points out that cloning has been shown to be unsafe, and there's no reason to suppose lab-created sperm will be any safer.

Still, all the experts say what has been done in Newcastle is interesting and good for research. Discovering how to make sperm will teach us more about sperm malfunction, and therefore could help treat infertile men, rather than replace them.

The Newcastle team used stem cells from a leftover embryo donated after fertility treatment, and used chemicals to encourage their growth. They could not use just any kind of stem cells, however. They selected only those with the potential to become sperm – the so-called 'germline' cells, which were a small proportion of the total.

The very notion that human sperm have been created from stem cells has taken anxieties to a new level

Over four to six weeks, these cells developed and were prompted to undergo the process of 'meiosis', which halved the number of chromosomes they carried – a hallmark of sperm. The woman's egg must contribute the rest of the chromosomes needed by an embryo.

Interestingly, the team's success came from stem cells with XY (male) chromosomes. The same process on XX (female) stem cells did not work, which seems to suggest that the male of the human species is not yet wholly superfluous.

9 July 2009

© Guardian News & Media Ltd 2009

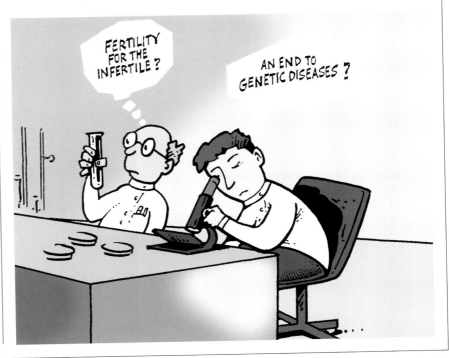

FERTILITY FOR THE INFERTILE?

AN END TO GENETIC DISEASES?

⇨ The first step in producing a new individual, fertilisation, can take place outside the body. In 1978, Louise Brown became the world's first 'test-tube baby'. Sperm and egg are fused in culture; the embryo develops a short while and is then implanted into the mother's womb. (page 1)

⇨ In the UK, about one in seven couples seek medical help to have a baby. (page 2)

⇨ Women in their early twenties are about twice as fertile as women in their late thirties. (page 4)

⇨ In Britain alone, 111,633 children have been born through fertility treatment; worldwide, the figure is estimated to be 3.5 million. (page 5)

⇨ The first IVF triplets were born in 1984. In recent years, the HFEA has raised concern over the relatively high incidence of multiple births conceived through IVF; the risk of death before birth or within the first week after birth is more than four times greater for twins, and almost seven times greater for triplets, than for single births. (page 6)

⇨ The first commercial surrogacy took place in Britain in 1985, when Kim Cotton, a mother of two, was paid £6,500 to carry a child conceived using her egg and the infertile woman's husband's sperm. It is now illegal for a surrogate to charge fees, but reasonable expenses may be paid. (page 7)

⇨ Britain is languishing behind other European countries in the number of IVF cycles provided for infertile couples and Brits are three times less likely to undergo IVF than those living in Denmark and Belgium, a study reveals. (page 8)

⇨ Most sperm donors are between the ages of 18-25 years and financial compensation seems to be the major motivation for donation. (page 11)

⇨ Until 2002 donor anonymity still existed in the UK. However, in 2004 the decision was taken that only sperm and egg donors who were willing to be identified at a later stage should be used, with effect from April 2005. (page 11)

⇨ An online survey of more than 300 fertility patients carried out for National Infertility Day has found that 76% would consider travelling overseas for their treatment. (page 18)

⇨ Most British IVF clinics will not offer services to women above the age of 50. The NHS will only provide fertility treatment up to the age of 40. (page 20)

⇨ Twins born as a result of assisted reproductive technology (ART) are more likely to be admitted to neonatal intensive care and to be hospitalised in their first three years of life than spontaneously conceived twins, according to new research. (page 21)

⇨ 54 per cent of NHS Primary Care Trusts exclude couples from IVF if one partner has a child from a previous relationship, leading to accusations that there is an IVF 'postcode lottery'. (page 22)

⇨ The number of women treated with donated sperm fell by about 20 per cent, from 2,727 in 2005 to 2,107 in 2006, the first full year after anonymity for sperm donors was removed. (page 24)

⇨ New research from Edinburgh University shows men who donated semen anonymously in the past are not necessarily comfortable with being unaware of the outcome of their donations. Many hope that life has turned out well for offspring created as a result of their donations. Some donors, it appears, hope that they may be traced by donor offspring and would then treat them as members of their family. (page 25)

⇨ Parents who have conceived children with the help of sperm or egg donors and then try to find the donors and also other children conceived with the donors' help, often end up creating new forms of extended families, according to new research. (page 26)

⇨ It's not new for doctors to use tissue from the brother or sister of a sick child in the hope of curing a serious disease. But since 2001, doctors have been able to test the cells of embryos created by IVF, to see whether they are a match for the sick child. This means that, in theory, parents could have babies they have chosen specifically to help their sick child. (page 28)

⇨ Since 1988 it has been shown that adult stem cells present in the blood of the umbilical cord can be used for transplantation in a number of genetic and blood diseases as well as immune deficiencies, e.g. leukaemia. After transplantation the stem cells repopulate the bone marrow of the patient, providing a source of blood cells. (page 33)

⇨ Using 'stem cells' from very early embryos (under 14 days of age), which are capable of developing into any of the specialised cells of the body, replacement tissue could be grown in the laboratory and used to cure many currently incurable conditions, avoiding the problem of immune rejection. But the use of human embryos raises ethical questions. (page 36)

GLOSSARY

ART
Assisted Reproduction Technologies. This refers to methods used to achieve pregnancy by artificial or partially artificial means.

'Designer baby'
Developments in pre-natal screening and IVF mean it is now hypothetically possible for parents to choose characteristics they would wish their child to have. While this may be used for medical reasons – for example, an embryo may be screened to find out if it will develop a life-limiting genetic disease – there are fears that some parents might try to use scientific advances to choose characteristics which they feel are cosmetically or socially desirable for their child, such as gender, athletic ability, IQ, hair or eye colour.

Donor
Someone who gives (donates) something to be used for someone else's benefit. Some people choose to donate their eggs and sperm in order to help infertile couples have children. Until relatively recently, they were able to do this anonymously: however, since April 2005 children conceived with donated gametes have had a legal right to find out the identity of their donor parent.

Embryo
A fertilised egg up until eight weeks after conception. After this time, it is referred to as a foetus. Some couples choose to have their embryos frozen so that they can be placed back into the womb and complete their development at a later date.

Embryonic stem cell
This type of stem cell is sometimes referred to as a 'building block' for the human body because it is completely unspecialised – it is capable of becoming any other cell type. These are very valuable to researchers trying to find treatments for certain illnesses. However, their use is also very controversial, with many pro-life groups deeply against the destruction of embryos for the purpose of 'harvesting' their cells. Stem cells used for research are typically obtained from 'waste' embryos created during the IVF process, with the consent of the donors.

Fertility
The ability to become pregnant or impregnate a partner. A couple may be diagnosed as having 'fertility problems' if they have been trying for a baby for a year without success.

Gametes
The cells which fuse together during reproduction (eggs and sperm).

IVF
In-Vitro Fertilisation – a process by which an egg can be fertilised outside of the human body. Sperm and egg are fused in culture; the embryo develops a short while and is then implanted into the mother's womb. Louise Brown was the first 'test-tube baby' created in this way in 1978.

Multiple births
IVF increases the risk of a multiple birth – twins, triplets or more – as several embryos may be implanted in the woman's womb at once. Implanting multiple embryos makes it more likely that at least one will 'take', but if a multiple pregnancy arises it will be more risky for mother and offspring than a pregnancy with a single baby.

Ovulation
The time during a woman's monthly cycle when an egg is released by the ovaries. This will usually happen in the middle of her cycle. A woman has the highest chance of becoming pregnant if she has sexual intercourse around this time. Ovulation problems are the most common cause of infertility in women.

Surrogacy
A situation where a woman agrees to have a child on behalf of someone else, either because the intended parents are infertile or for some other reason. Straight surrogacy is when the host mother uses her own egg and is artificially inseminated with the sperm of the intended father. Gestational or host surrogacy occurs when the egg of the intended mother and sperm of the intended father are used. The surrogate (host) mother will not therefore be biologically related to the child. However, by UK law she is still considered the child's mother until the intended parents can legally adopt the baby. In the UK, it is illegal to be paid for surrogacy, but a certain amount of money can be given to cover expenses.

'Saviour sibling'
Doctors are now able to screen embryos created by IVF to see if their cells are a match for a sick sibling. Parents can therefore choose to have a new baby so that his or her umbilical cord cells can be used to cure an illness suffered by an existing child. Babies created for this reason are often referred to as 'saviour siblings', because they may be able to save the life of their sick brother or sister.

INDEX

Additional Resources

Other Issues *titles*
If you are interested in researching further some of the issues raised in *Reproductive Ethics*, you may like to read the following titles in the **Issues** series:

⇨ Vol. 171 *Abortion – Rights and Ethics* (ISBN 978 1 86168 485 1)

⇨ Vol. 169 *The Animal Rights Debate* (ISBN 978 1 86168 473 8)

⇨ Vol. 152 *Euthanasia and the Right to Die* (ISBN 978 1 86168 439 4)

⇨ Vol. 148 *Religious Beliefs* (ISBN 978 1 86168 421 9)

⇨ Vol. 144 *The Cloning Debate* (ISBN 978 1 86168 410 3)

⇨ Vol. 138 *A Genetically-Modified Future?* (ISBN 978 1 86168 390 8)

⇨ Vol. 135 *Coping with Disability* (ISBN 978 1 86168 387 8)

For more information about these titles, visit our website at www.independence.co.uk/publicationslist

Useful organisations
You may find the websites of the following organisations useful for further research:

⇨ **BioCentre:** www.bioethics.ac.uk

⇨ **BioNews:** www.bionews.org.uk

⇨ **British Humanist Association:** www.humanism.org.uk

⇨ **British Medical Journal:** www.bmj.com

⇨ **Channel 4:** www.channel4.com

⇨ **The Christian Institute:** www.christian.org.uk

⇨ **Comment on Reproductive Ethics:** www.corethics.org

⇨ **Economic and Social Research Council:** www.esrc.ac.uk

⇨ **European Society of Human Reproduction and Embryology:** www.eshre.com

⇨ **Infertility Network UK:** www.infertilitynetworkuk.com

⇨ **Irish Council for Bioethics:** www.bioethics.i.e.

⇨ **NHS Choices:** www.nhs.uk

⇨ **The Wellcome Trust:** www.wellcome.ac.uk

⇨ **Women's Health:** www.womens-health.co.uk

ACKNOWLEDGEMENTS

The publisher is grateful for permission to reproduce the following material.

While every care has been taken to trace and acknowledge copyright, the publisher tenders its apology for any accidental infringement or where copyright has proved untraceable. The publisher would be pleased to come to a suitable arrangement in any such case with the rightful owner.

Chapter One: Making Babies

Doing without sex, © Big Picture Publications, *Fertility problems*, © BMJ Publishing Group Limited, *Causes of infertility*, © Crown copyright is reproduced with the permission of Her Majesty's Stationery Office, *IVF: the birth that started a revolution*, © Telegraph Media Group Limited (2009), *UK lags behind the rest of Europe in IVF*, © BioNews, *Having children for same-sex couples*, © Crown copyright is reproduced with the permission of Her Majesty's Stationery Office, *Egg and sperm donation*, © BioCentre, *Addicted to surrogacy*, © Telegraph Media Group Limited (2009), *Surrogacy*, © Women's Health, *Adoption in the UK*, © Infertility Network UK.

Chapter Two: Ethical Dilemmas

The 'test-tube baby' at 30, © Guardian News & Media Ltd 2009, *Fertility tourism*, © Infertility Network UK, *Is 66 too old to have a baby?*, © Telegraph Media Group Limited (2009), *Health problems for IVF twins*, © European Society of Human Reproduction and Embryology, *No end to IVF 'postcode lottery'*, © Channel 4, *Winston: egg freezing is 'expensive confidence trick'*, © BioNews, *The donor crisis*, © Times Newspapers Ltd, *Sperm donors are curious too*, © Economic and Social Research Council, *Donors creating new forms of extended families*, © European Society of Reproduction and Embryology, *'Saviour siblings'*, © BMJ Publishing Group, *My Jamie is not a 'designer baby'...*, © Guardian News & Media Ltd 2009, *Row over clinic that offers eye, skin and hair colour*, © Telegraph Media Group Limited (2009), *Stem cell research: hope or hype?*, © Irish Council for Bioethics, *Pope slams embryo research as immoral*, © Christian Institute, *A humanist discussion of embryo research*, © British Humanist Association, *Victory for ethics?*, © Comment on Reproductive Ethics (CORE), *Can sperm really be created in a laboratory?*, © Guardian News & Media Ltd 2009.

Photographs

Stock Xchng: pages 11 (Emily Cahal); 19 (melbia); 23a (Billy Alexander); 25 (Helmut Gevert); 28 (Lonnie Bradley); 31 (tim & annette).
Wikimedia Commons: pages 3, 23b, 35 (public domain); 36, 38 (this image was published in a Public Library of Science journal: *Follow the Money – The Politics of Embryonic Stem Cell Research*. Russo E, PLoS Biology Vol. 3/7/2005, e234 http://dx.doi.org/10.1371/journal.pbio.0030234).

Illustrations

Pages 1, 24, 33: Angelo Madrid; pages 4, 12, 27, 37: Simon Kneebone; pages 7, 13: Bev Aisbett; pages 9, 21, 30, 39: Don Hatcher.

And with thanks to the team: Mary Chapman, Sandra Dennis, Claire Owen and Jan Sunderland.

Lisa Firth
Cambridge
September, 2009